Shared Care for
Breast Disease

Shared Care for
Breast Disease

Family practitioners and hospital specialists
working together to improve patient care

by
Professor Samuel J. Leinster BSc MD FRCS
Professor of Surgery and Director of Medical Studies,
The University of Liverpool, UK

Dr Trevor J. Gibbs MB ChB MMedSci FFHom FRCGP
Director of Community Teaching, Department of Primary
Care, The University of Liverpool, UK

Ms Hilary Downey BSc RGN MPhil
Breast Care Specialist Nurse, Breast Assessment Unit,
Royal Liverpool University Hospital, UK

I S I S
MEDICAL
M E D I A

© 2000 by Isis Medical Media Ltd.
59 St Aldates
Oxford OX1 1ST, UK

First published 2000

British Library Cataloguing-in-Publication Data.
A catalogue record for this title is available
from the British Library.

ISBN 1 901865 57 6

Leinster, S.J. (Samuel)
Shared Care for Breast Disease
Samuel J. Leinster, Trevor J. Gibbs, Hilary Downey (eds)

Always refer to the manufacturer's Prescribing
Information before prescribing drugs cited in this book.

Medical art
Adrian and Gudrun Cornford

Design, illustrations and typesetting
In Perspective Ltd.

Indexing
Kathleen Lyle

1 0 0 4 6 0 4 6 7 8

Isis Medical Media staff
Commissioning Editor: Jonathan Gregory
Senior Editorial Controller: Sarah Carlson
Production & Editorial Manager: Julia Savory

Printed and bound by
Sun Fung Offset Bindings Co. Ltd., Printed in China

Distributed in the USA by
Books International, Inc., P.O. Box 605,
Herndon, VA 20172, USA

Distributed in the rest of the world by
Plymbridge Distributors Ltd., Estover Road,
Plymouth PL6 7PY, UK

Contents

Preface

Women are understandably anxious when they develop symptoms relating to the breast. The attempts over recent years to raise awareness of breast disease through health promotion campaigns have been successful and have resulted in large numbers of women presenting to their primary care teams. The patients' expectations have been raised and many will wish to be referred to specialist units. The general practitioner is faced with difficult decisions on management. Should the patient be referred? What investigation or treatment is appropriate?

When women have undergone treatment for breast cancer there is a tendency for the specialist units to take over care completely and, intentionally or unintentionally, to exclude the primary care team. Is this in the best interests of the patient?

It is clear that a better understanding between the primary and secondary care teams is needed if the patients are to get the best deal. This book is written with the aim of improving that understanding.

Sam Leinster is a surgeon with a special interest in breast disease. He developed the Breast Unit in the Royal Liverpool University Hospital from a single consultant surgeon and a radiologist seeing 50 new cancers a year to a multidisciplinary team seeing almost 400 new cancers a year. He is still actively engaged in the management of breast disease. Trevor Gibbs is an experienced General Practitioner. Hilary Downey was a Research Assistant in the Breast Unit carrying out studies in breast pain and benign breast disease. She is now one of the team of four Breast Care Nurses on the unit.

The case presentations and discussions are real. Dr Chris Thomas who is a local General Practitioner joined the authors for the discussions and we are grateful for her contribution. The discussions do read, rather unfortunately, like an old-style tutorial with the tutor dispensing wisdom, but they are a faithful recounting of our actual conversations. The initials of the discussant are given with each of their contributions and should be self-evident to the reader.

The management of breast cancer is increasingly evidence based and is rapidly evolving. We have attempted to set out principles rather than detail. We hope that this will provide a basis for a dialogue between the primary care team and the cancer specialists that will result in improved care for the patients.

Professor Samuel J. Leinster
Dr Trevor J. Gibbs
Ms Hilary Downey
Liverpool, UK, 1999

chapter 1

The background to breast disease

EPIDEMIOLOGY

The increased public awareness of breast problems, the increasingly extensive media coverage and the Government decision to include breast cancer as one of the main areas of its *Health of the Nation* policy have meant that diseases of the breast occupy an increasing amount of medical time and activity. With the changing incidence of breast cancer and the possible association with modern medical management, breast disorders could be classed as a relatively new problem. However, the subject appears to occupy a large place in medical history. From as early as the first century AD, medical scholars were writing about the value of cautery to resolve malignant breast lumps. Distinguished authors such as Hippocrates and Celsus wrote extensively upon the clinical aspects of breast disease, while Galen described the surgical and conservative management of breast disorders as early as 130AD. But how important and how common is breast disease in modern health care?

Breast disorders account for a large number of general practice consultations; about 30 new patients per 1000 women seen every year by a general practitioner (GP) have a breast problem. This does not reflect those consultations in which breast problems are mentioned as an aside or as a minor complaint as part of any other screening, health promotion or problem-led encounter. In the UK, approximately 230 000 women with breast abnormalities are referred to hospital each year. Fortunately, only just less than 6% of referrals from general practice culminate in a diagnosis of breast cancer. The nature of breast disorders and the difficulties experienced in making an accurate diagnosis have resulted in an increased referral rate to hospitals, especially in the age group 20–40 years for which the referral rate has increased by 80%.

In a general surgical unit, breast problems can occupy at least 25% of the workload. There are many different presentations (Fig. 1.1), but the majority of women complain of a lump.

Epidemiological studies of breast disease have tended to concentrate on breast cancer, even though only 10% of women who attend a breast clinic are eventually given a diagnosis of breast cancer. Some 50% of women in the UK will have a problem with their breast at some time in their reproductive life. The management of benign breast disease is discussed in a later chapter, but the incidence of certain benign breast disorders is discussed here (Fig. 1.2).

Congenital breast problems and *variations on the norm* are common. Supernumerary and accessory nipples and aberrant breast tissue are found

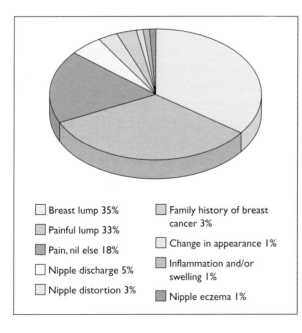

Breast lump 35%

Painful lump 33%

Pain, nil else 18%

Nipple discharge 5%

Nipple distortion 3%

Family history of breast cancer 3%

Change in appearance 1%

Inflammation and/or swelling 1%

Nipple eczema 1%

Figure 1.1.
Presentations of breast disease. Breast disease presents in a variety of ways. More than half of the women who present experience pain, and a lump is present in almost 70%. Although self-examination leaflets emphasize nipple discharge and change of shape, these symptoms are comparatively uncommon.

in between 1 and 5% of the population. Individuals frequently present to the GP from whom reassurance is the mainstay of management.

Although some degree of breast asymmetry is common, it is possible to have either a hypoplastic or completely absent breast that requires augmentation. Often associated with breast asymmetry and hypoplasia are defects in the pectoral muscles of the anterior chest wall.

Normal physiological changes in the breast often lead to consultation. Unilateral enlargement of the pubertal female breast causes concern, particularly if associated with pain and discomfort. Uncontrolled overgrowth of breast tissue can occur in adolescent girls with a normal

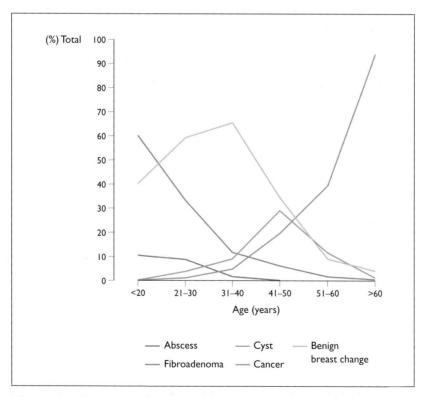

Figure 1.2. Percentage of patients with discrete breast lumps who have given condition (by age).

hormonal profile, and is sometimes severe enough to warrant reduction mammoplasty to save social embarrassment.

Gynaecomastia is common in boys during puberty, occurring in 30–60% of boys between 10–16 years of age. Idiopathic or senescent gynaecomastia can occur in men between 60–80 years of age, but is a diagnosis of exclusion after more important causes have been eliminated.

Fibroadenomas account for about 12% of all palpable breast lumps and are particularly common in the age group 15–30 years. In females under 20 years of age, fibroadenomas account for approximately 60% of breast lumps. Although 5% of fibroadenomas grow progressively, 20% regress in the short term. The majority stay the same size until the menopause and regress thereafter.

Benign breast cysts are commonly found in a later age group (40–50 years). They are frequently multiple, often asymptomatic and often found accidentally by the patient.

Breast pain is experienced by most women at some time in their reproductive life; 66% of working women and 77% of any screened population have breast pain severe enough to mention. There are three main types of breast pain (mastalgia). The most common is cyclical mastalgia, which accounts for 75% of all cases. Non-cyclical mastalgia is less common, has no relationship to the menstrual cycle, occurs in an older population and resolves spontaneously in 50% of cases. The third group of breast pain is musculoskeletal pain arising from structures adjacent to the breasts. The commonest form of this is Tietze's syndrome which is costochondritis of the underlying rib.

Breast cancer

Breast cancer accounts for 18% of all female cancer deaths in the UK and, other than in certain areas of Scotland and North-West England, is still the most common cause of death from any cancer (Fig. 1.3).

World-wide there are 57 000 new cases per year. In the UK, where the age-standardized incidence and mortality is the highest in the world, the incidence among women of age 50 years approaches 2/100 per year. In the UK, 4000 new cases occur per year in women less than

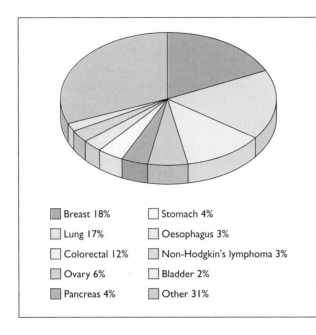

Figure 1.3.
Cancer deaths in women in the UK in 1995 (data from the Cancer Research Campaign Scientific Yearbook, 1995).

Breast 18%   Stomach 4%

Lung 17%   Oesophagus 3%

Colorectal 12% Non-Hodgkin's lymphoma 3%

Ovary 6%   Bladder 2%

Pancreas 4%   Other 31%

45 years of age. There are 15 000 deaths per year and the incidence is increasing by about 1–2% per year. In women 50 years of age, 20/1000 will develop breast cancer; 15/1000 have had breast cancer diagnosed before the age of 50 years, which gives an overall prevalence of approximately 3.5%.

Between the years of 1950 and 1970 mortality from breast cancer in England and Wales increased by 16% in women aged 15–44 years. Since the 1980s, the breast cancer death rate has continued to fall. This decrease is greater for younger women and may represent a better detection service and improved management regimes.

Risk factors for breast cancer

Family history Between 5 and 10% of breast cancers in western society have a genetic component. The mode of inheritance is believed to be autosomal dominant and of variable penetrance. Around 50% of inherited breast cancer is thought to result from an abnormal gene on the long arm of chromosome 17, *BRCA1*, while others result from an abnormal gene found on the long arm of chromosome 13, *BRCA2*. There is an association with other neoplasia, particularly colon, prostate and ovary.

Certain ethic groups are more susceptible, notably Ashkenazi Jews carrying the *BRCA1* mutation.

A woman's risk of breast cancer is twice as great if she has a first-degree relative who developed breast cancer before 50 years of age.

Age Breast cancer incidence increases with age and doubles every 10 years until menopause (Fig. 1.4). After 50 years of age the rate of increase of the incidence slows. Expressed in another way, in women younger than 35 the cumulative risk of developing breast cancer is 1 in 625. At age 50 years the cumulative risk is 1 in 56, at 60 it is 1 in 18 and at 75 it is 1 in 13.

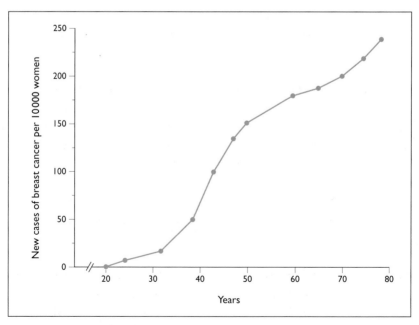

Figure 1.4. Age-related incidence of breast cancer.

Medical history The cancer risk associated with benign breast disease is low, probably less than a two-fold increase over women with no history of breast disease. Severe atypical epithelial hyperplasia increases the chance of breast cancer four-fold. Women with duct papillomas, palpable cysts and the more complex fibroadenomas have twice the risk of breast cancer.

Previous exposure to radiation There is evidence that high levels of radiation to the breast increase the risk of developing breast cancer. This risk is highest when the radiation occurs during adolescence. The benefits derived from mammography far outweigh any potential increase in the incidence of breast cancer in women over 40 years of age.

Gynaecological factors An early menarche and a late onset of the menopause are both associated with an increased risk of breast cancer. Nulliparity and late age at first birth are both risk factors. Women who have their first child after 30 years of age carry twice the risk of breast cancer compared to women who have their first child before 20 years of age. Protection derived from pregnancy only applies if the pregnancy goes to term.

Geographical variation As society changes and indigenous populations change, the variation between the incidence of breast cancer throughout the world becomes less. However, the difference in breast cancer between Asian nations and Western nations is still five-fold. There are likely to be a number of reasons for this variation.

Life style No association appears to occur between breast cancer and alcohol and smoking, although obesity is associated with a two-fold increase.

Exogenous hormones Various national and international studies have failed collectively to agree as to the association between breast cancer and taking oral contraceptives (the Pill). If all women who have taken the Pill, regardless of age, parity, family history, etc., are studied, no increased risk of breast cancer is found. However, those women currently taking or who have recently stopped taking the Pill have a 25% increase in relative risk. This increased risk decreases with time and is absent after 10 years of stopping the Pill.

The relationship between hormonal replacement therapy (HRT) and breast cancer is also debatable. Studies of women taking unopposed oestrogen show that the relative risk of breast cancer increases by up to 50% after 10–15 years of continuous use. The benefits of taking HRT, however, outweigh the potential risks for the first 10 years of use.

BIOLOGY

The adult female breast is made up of 15–20 lobes covered with a variable amount of adipose tissue. Each lobe contains several secretory lobules that give rise to ducts. The ducts from all the lobules in a single lobe converge into a single lactiferous duct that opens individually on the surface of the nipple through a lactiferous sinus (Fig. 1.5).

Breast cancer develops from the epithelial cells of the terminal ducts. It is generally thought that a sequence of gradual changes occurs from the normal cell to invasive carcinoma (Fig. 1.6). This is governed by a series of mutations in the genes. A further genetic change is needed before the tumour acquires the ability to metastasize. In colonic cancer the sequence of genetic events has been clearly worked out, but this is not the case for breast cancer.

GENETICS

Only 5–10% of breast cancer is hereditary, but all breast cancer is a result of mutations within the breast cells. A number of genetic abnormalities identified in breast tumours can be used to estimate the prognosis for a given tumour. As yet, the role of these genetic abnormalities in the development of breast cancer is not clear. Three classes of genes

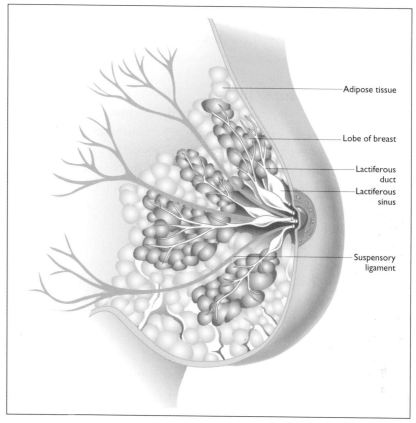

Figure 1.5. The anatomy of the breast.

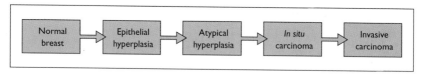

Figure 1.6. The development of breast cancer.

have been suggested to have a role in the aetiology of breast cancer – oncogenes, tumour suppressor genes and genes that determine metastatic potential. The genes that control the expression of receptors and of cell adhesion molecules may also be mutated and affect the prognosis.

Oncogenes

Oncogenes are genes that have a role in the control of the cell cycle. When these genes are mutated, the control of cell growth is lost.

Tumour suppressor genes

Tumour suppressor genes are also part of the normal regulatory mechanism that control the cell cycle. The most common tumour suppressor gene that is mutated in breast cancer is *p53*, which codes for a protein involved in the control of the cell cycle. Normal (wild type) *p53* is activated when abnormalities occur in DNA transcription. The cell cycle is arrested and the cell undergoes apoptosis, or programmed cell death, thus preventing replication of the abnormal DNA. When mutant *p53* replaces the wild type, this process does not take place and the abnormal DNA continues to replicate, which gives rise to cancer cells. Tumours that contain mutant *p53* have a worse prognosis than tumours that do not.

Mutations in the *BRCA1* and *BRCA2* tumour suppressor genes are less common than those in *p53*, but are important because these genes have been identified as responsible for familial breast cancer. They are present at low frequency in the general population, but are more common in certain populations such as the Ashkenazi Jews.

Metastasis genes

Even when a tumour has become invasive, it may lack metastatic potential. Mutations in genes such as *nm23* and *p9ka* are needed before metastases can occur.

Genes that control growth factor and steroid receptors

The importance of oestrogen and progesterone receptors in determining the behaviour of the tumours has been recognized for a long time. When functioning receptors are present, the tumour has a better prognosis, and this is not just related to its increased responsiveness to hormone treatment. Receptors for growth factors such as epithelial growth factor (EGF) are present on the cell surface. A number of growth factor receptors are now recognized, including some such as *c-erbB2* for which the ligand has yet to be identified. When the growth factors are over-expressed, the prognosis of the tumour is poorer.

Genes that control cell adhesion molecules

The normal stability of tissues is maintained by adhesion between cells and by the contact inhibition of growth. Mutations of the molecules involved in these processes (cathepsins, cadherins and integrins) have been recognized. These mutations are associated with a poorer prognosis.

The different patterns of mutations within tumours presumably account in part for the difference in behaviour of the tumours.

PATHOLOGY OF BREAST DISEASE

The aetiology of benign breast disease is poorly understood. Clinically, the most common finding is a painful or tender lumpy breast. The histological findings in these cases range from normal breast tissue to fibrosis, adenosis and microcyst formation. These may be described by the pathologist as fibroadenosis or fibrocystic disease, but are probably best described by the rather nondescript term benign breast change, which emphasizes that these findings are variants of normal rather than true disease states. At one time it was thought that these changes were risk factors for breast cancer. It is now clear that the increased risk is related to certain specific changes, in particular *atypical epithelial hyperplasia*.

Breast cysts are part of this spectrum of disease. Two distinct types are recognized – apocrine cysts (Fig. 1.7a) and flattened epithelial cysts. The former have an associated increased risk of the development of breast cancer, but this is not sufficiently strong to warrant regular follow-up of women with cysts unless the cysts are multiple and recurrent.

Fibroadenomas (Fig. 1.7b) have in the past been regarded as benign tumours of the breast, but it is likely that they are aberrations of the normal cycle of development and involution. They do not have any malignant potential and do not need to be removed unless they are enlarging.

Phylloides tumour (which used to be known somewhat confusingly as cystosarcoma phylloides) is a rare tumour that is usually benign in its behaviour, although it has a propensity to recur locally after removal. A few are genuinely malignant and metastasize. It is difficult to predict on morphological grounds which phylloides tumours will do this.

Duct ectasia is common and is associated with ageing. It may give rise to *periductal mastitis*, which is also found in younger women who smoke. The mechanism that underlies this association is unclear. Periductal mastitis is usually the result of an anaerobic infection and may progress to abscess formation or *mammary duct fistula*.

Breast cancer (Fig. 1.7c) is an adenocarcinoma. *In situ* carcinoma may be ductal (DCIS; Fig. 1.7d) or lobular (LCIS); the latter is probably best regarded as a marker of increased risk for breast cancer. Over a 10-year follow-up period, the risk of the development of an invasive breast cancer in a woman in whom LCIS has been found is about 30%. There is an equal chance of the cancer appearing in either breast. In contrast, DCIS is considered to be a pre-invasive stage of breast cancer. The risk of recurrence after treatment depends on the grade and type of DCIS.

The majority of invasive carcinomas (75%) are classified as ductal carcinomas of no special type, 10–15% are infiltrating lobular carcinomas and the remainder are carcinomas of special type (tubular, papillary, medullary), which have a better prognosis than the more common tumours. Tumours of no special type are graded on the basis of their histological characteristics – Grade 1 tumours are well-differentiated, Grade 3 are poorly differentiated and Grade 2 are intermediate.

Breast cancer is generally slow growing and the preclinical phase may be up to 8 years long. Metastases can occur before the tumour is clinically palpable. The classic view of breast cancer was that it spread in a centrifugal fashion. The tumour entered the lymphatics and spread first to the lower axillary lymph nodes. It then progressed up the lymph nodes before entering the bloodstream and spreading to distant parts of the body (Fig. 1.8a). This was the rationale behind the use of radical mastectomy, which removed the breast and all the axillary lymph nodes. More recently, breast cancer has been regarded as a disease that

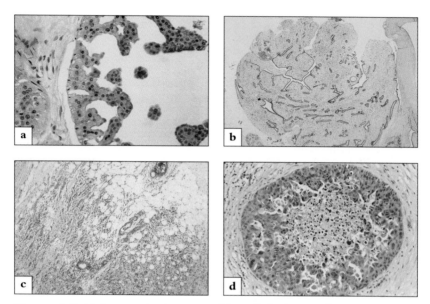

Figure 1.7. (a) An apocrine breast cyst. The cellular lining of this cyst is more florid than usual and is developing a papillary pattern. (b) A typical benign fibroadenoma. (c) Typical invasive carcinoma of the breast. Note the cancer cells infiltrating the fatty stroma. (d) Intraduct carcinoma (DCIS) of comedo type. Note the central area of necrosis. The cells look malignant but are contained within the basement membrane of the duct. Calcification may occur within the area of necrosis and thus render the DCIS visible on mammography.

is systemic from a very early stage. The cancer cells enter the blood-stream directly from the tumour and do not have to pass through the lymph nodes first (Fig. 1.8b).

PROGNOSIS OF BREAST CANCER

As a general rule, the earlier a breast cancer is detected, the better is the prognosis. Prediction of prognosis depends on the size of the tumour, the extent of lymph node involvement and the biological characteristics of the tumour (whether it is aggressive or not). There

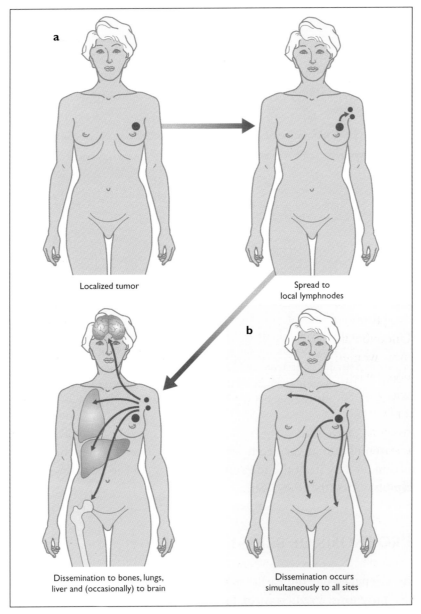

Localized tumor

Spread to
local lymphnodes

Dissemination to bones, lungs,
liver and (occasionally) to brain

Dissemination occurs
simultaneously to all sites

Figure 1.8. (a) Centrifugal theory of breast cancer metastasis. (b) Current view of breast cancer metastasis.

are a number of biological markers for the latter property, including the various gene products mentioned above, but the one commonly used is grade. The higher the grade the worse the prognosis. These factors can be incorporated into a prognostic index, the most commonly used of which is the Nottingham index (Equation 1.1).

EQUATION 1.1 $\text{PI} = 0.2 \times \text{size (cm)} + \text{nodal status} + \text{grade}$

Equation 1.1 gives a numerical score, which can be related to tables that predict the outcome. Treatment decisions may be based on the prognostic information that is obtained (Fig. 1.9).

PSYCHOLOGY

Most women who present with breast lumps (or, indeed, any other breast symptom such as nipple discharge) are emotionally distressed. Undoubtedly, these women fear they may have breast cancer. Although most women who seek advice from their doctor are eventually diagnosed with a benign breast disorder or no disease at all, some of those with benign disorders remain clinically depressed. While there have been a plethora of studies into psychological factors and breast cancer, relatively few have been conducted in patients with benign breast disease. Clearly, more studies for this group are needed.

Benign breast disorders

Studies have been carried out on women presenting to a breast clinic with either a palpable breast lump or a nipple discharge. It has been found that severe depression is more common in those women found to have benign breast disorders than those subsequently diagnosed with breast cancer. The depression was thought to be associated with recent life events and social difficulties.

Similarly, mood changes that have been found in women complaining of moderate cyclical mastalgia are thought to offer an explanation

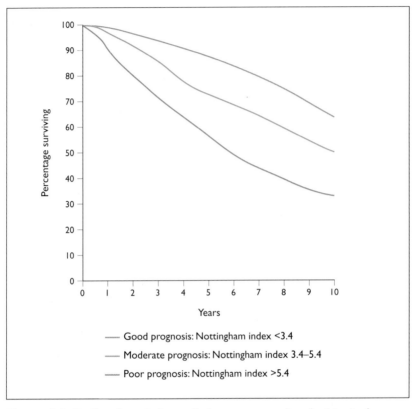

Figure 1.9. Predicted survival rates for breast cancer using the Nottingham prognostic index. (NB: These figures relate to women who are not receiving adjuvant treatment. The odds of death are reduced by approximately 30% at 10 years for all women who receive adjuvant therapy. The survival for the good prognosis group would be ~80% if adjuvants were given.)

as to why some women seek treatment and others do not. This observation is particularly interesting because mastalgia is an underreported condition. Two studies showed mastalgia to have a high incidence (68.9% and 66%, respectively), but only a minority of women had sought treatment (3.4% and 10%, respectively).

High levels of anxiety and depression have been observed in women who report severe cyclical mastalgia. The psychological distress of these patients has been found to be similar to that experienced by women on the morning of their definitive surgery for breast cancer. Furthermore, even when severe breast pain was successfully treated (by hormonal manipulations), anxiety was reduced but not fully resolved, whereas depression was relieved along with breast symptoms. High-anxiety proneness was also identified in this group.

Likewise, high levels of anxiety have been found in other cases of benign breast disorder. One study suggested that the highest levels were found in new patients presenting with cysts.

However, women recalled from the breast screening programme have high levels of anxiety as a result of their concerns about the possibility of breast cancer rather than a possible underlying psychological problem.

Breast cancer

It has been estimated that as many as 30% of patients newly diagnosed with breast cancer develop an anxiety or depressive illness within a year of diagnosis.

Unfortunately, many patients feel unable to disclose this psychological morbidity because they think it is of no interest to the health-care team. The health-care team can help by asking questions about how the patient is feeling about the nature of their illness and reactions to treatments, which will encourage disclosure of feelings. For some women, morbidity continues after the diagnosis is known and following treatment. Those women who do not return to normal function need to be identified, so that appropriate help can be offered and initiated.

Treatments for breast cancer may lead to psychological morbidity. It has been suggested that the use of wide local excision (with breast conservation) rather than mastectomy may reduce psychological morbidity caused by surgery. However, this may not always be so. Reconstruction following mastectomy is an alternative approach to preserving body image. While many women who choose reconstruction are comforted by their result and do not experience the constant reminder (mastectomy site) of their breast cancer, for some women it is ineffective. Those who have had complications from their reconstructive surgery or who obtain a poor cosmetic result may have increased difficulties adapting to their body image.

Patients undergoing chemotherapy may experience physical and emotional problems. Many suffer side effects of hair loss, weight gain, skin changes, nausea and vomiting, diarrhoea, sore mouth, food cravings and menopausal symptoms. These effects do little to enhance body image. However, women tolerate these symptoms in the hope that the treatment will keep the cancer at bay (adjuvant treatment) or will reduce the unwanted symptoms of advanced disease (e.g. breathlessness caused by lung metastases).

Endocrine therapies may also evoke some unwanted side effects (hot flushes, weight gain, nausea, vaginal bleeding or dryness, lethargy). Some women find these symptoms quite distressing and need a sympathetic approach to controlling these side effects.

For those women prone to claustrophobia, the need for radiotherapy could be distressing; and they may experience panic attacks at the thought of being in a small room while receiving treatment. Body image may be altered by skin reactions to radiotherapy and altered breast size in some cases.

These side effects of treatments may have an impact upon sexual relationships, either because of emotional problems associated with treatments, or as a direct result of the treatment on the female hormones (and hence femininity also); or by simply feeling less attractive. Sexual problems are often multifactorial and need sensitive and supportive listening to allow women to express their feelings. Where appropriate, advice, symptom control or referral to specialist help may be useful.

SCREENING FOR BREAST CANCER

Since there is no known primary prevention for breast cancer, secondary prevention in the form of breast screening has been introduced in an attempt to reduce mortality from the disease. The only screening method proved to result in reduction of mortality is regular mammography; this is the method used in the National Health Service Breast Screening Programme in the UK. Current screening programmes for breast cancer do not fully meet the principles of screening set out by the World Health Organization (see box below), as the screening test is comparatively expensive in monetary terms and requires highly skilled medical and technical staff who are in short supply. Despite this, the majority of expert opinion favours the adoption of mammographic screening, as it has been shown to reduce mortality.

Other forms of screening, such as clinical examination and breast self-examination, are a matter of controversy. Some series suggest that the addition of clinical examination to mammography improves the detection rate. It has yet to be shown that this results in any improvement in survival. In the developing world, the introduction of a programme of breast self-examination may result in presentation of breast cancer at an earlier stage, with a consequent improvement in survival, but this effect is not seen in the developed world.

PRINCIPLES OF SCREENING

- The disease being screened for must be common and important

- There must be an efficient, cost-effective and acceptable method of detecting the disease at an early stage

- There must be an effective treatment for the disease

- Early treatment must produce a better outcome than later treatment

If screening is to make an impact on survival it must be *sensitive*; that is, it must detect the majority of cancers that exist. This means that a number of benign abnormalities (false positives) will be detected and diagnosis must be made as quickly and accurately as possible to avoid unnecessary anxiety among the women who are screened. If steps are taken to make the test more *specific* so that more of the abnormalities detected are, in fact, breast cancer, more false negatives will occur and treatable cancers will be missed. There is inevitably a trade-off between sensitivity and specificity.

Any screening programme must make arrangements for the rapid assessment and diagnosis of women who are found to have abnormalities. Ideally, the same team should be involved from screening through to treatment.

CHAPTER SUMMARY

- Breast disease is the most common cancer in women in the UK
- Most women with breast symptoms do not have breast cancer
- The development of breast cancer is the result of changes in the molecular genetics of the cells
- The prognosis of breast cancer is dependent on the interaction of a number of factors; some breast cancers have an extremely good prognosis.

chapter 2

Presentations of breast disease

The presentation of breast disease is limited. There are basically four complaints – a lump, pain, discharge or distortion of the breast. More rarely, rashes that affect the nipple may present a diagnostic challenge.

LUMP

The most common presentation is a lump. Many of the patients who complain of a lump have lumpiness rather than a true lump. The distinction between the two is a matter of clinical judgement and can be difficult. Traditionally, lumps can be felt with the flat of the finger-tips, whereas lumpiness feels like a lump only when it is held between finger and thumb. It is better to err on the side of safety and consider lumpiness to be a lump that needs investigation rather than to dismiss a true lump without investigation. Whether lumpiness indicates an increased risk of the development of breast cancer depends on the nature of the underlying pathology.

Lumps can be differentiated from lumpiness on the basis of the history. Lumpiness tends to vary with the menstrual cycle, whereas lumps do not. A clear history of trauma might indicate that the lump is a haematoma or an area of fat necrosis, but mild trauma might draw the attention of the patient to a pre-existing carcinoma. A history of trauma does not exclude carcinoma. When doubt exists it is useful to re-examine the breast at a different phase of the menstrual cycle to determine whether the palpable abnormality has changed. A family history of breast cancer or a personal past history of breast disease may give a woman greater breast awareness. This results in a higher likelihood of presentation, but is of no help in the diagnosis of the lump.

Lumpiness tends to affect the upper, outer quadrant of the breast, but this is also the most common site for true lumps. Bilateral palpable abnormalities are more likely to be lumpiness than true lumps, but beware the women with lumpy breasts who develops a new discrete lump on one side.

The likely diagnosis of a discrete lump in the breast depends on the age of the patient (see Fig 1.2):

- 15–30 years, fibroadenoma
- 30–50 years, cyst
- 40+ years, carcinoma.

These age-based diagnoses are not absolute, and the diagnosis should be based on the nature of the lump and not on the age of the patient.

While expert clinical examination results in the accurate diagnosis of about 95% of breast cancers, a definitive diagnosis of a lump can be made only by using the *triple assessment* approach (see Chapter 3).

PAIN (MASTALGIA)

Mastalgia is the most common breast symptom reported to the GP. Historically, mastalgia was regarded as a trivial complaint with psychological origins for which little could be done; however, it has been shown that these women are not neurotic and deserve a therapeutic approach to the management of their symptoms. Intriguingly, it is an under-reported symptom despite the significant impact on the lifestyle of some women.

Breast pain can be classified into three categories – cyclical, non-cyclical and non-breast.

Cyclical mastalgia

The breast discomfort of cyclical mastalgia occurs in conjunction with the menstrual cycle. It is experienced during the reproductive years of a woman's life and disappears after the menopause. Many women experience some breast discomfort for a few days premenstrually, but cyclical mastalgia is said to be present when the symptoms are pronounced – they are experienced for longer during the cycle and are more severe (Fig. 2.1). Typically, the pain is absent (or at its mildest) during the follicular phase of the menstrual cycle and it is maximal during the luteal phase. The symptoms usually subside with the onset of the next menstrual cycle. (The symptoms wax and wane with each cycle.) Some women may complain of symptoms for most of their cycle that worsen premenstrually and some women are never pain free.

Typically, the pain is diffuse, but most frequently is reported to affect the upper outer quadrant of the breast. Nodularity may (but may not always) be felt on palpation during the clinical examination of the breasts. The pain may be experienced in one breast only, in both breasts, or it may radiate down the ipsilateral arm.

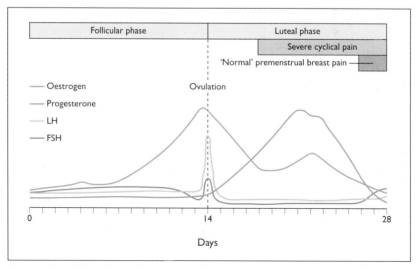

Figure 2.1. The relationship of cyclical mastalgia to the menstrual cycle.

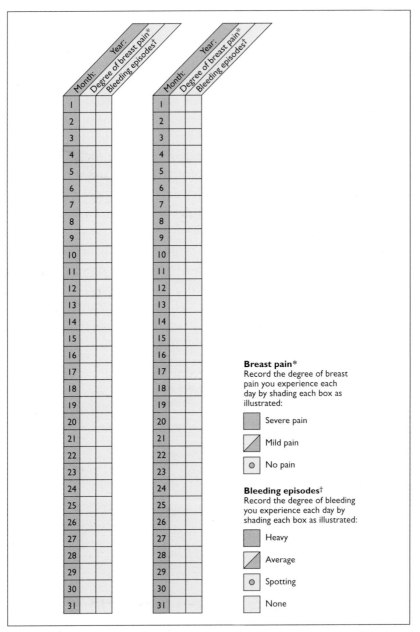

Figure 2.2. Daily breast-pain chart.

Women who seek treatment for cyclical mastalgia may have experienced symptoms from as little as 1 month before presentation to considerably longer (several years in some cases). Relief from symptoms may occur spontaneously (22% of cases in one study), and usually follows a hormonal event such as pregnancy, use of oral contraceptives or the menopause. While some women may respond well to an explanation of the symptoms with reassurance that the pain is not associated with a breast cancer, many women have symptoms sufficiently severe to warrant treatment.

The cyclical nature of the symptoms is usually confirmed by completion of a diary chart (Fig. 2.2), even for women who have had a hysterectomy with preservation of ovaries.

Cyclical pain (Fig. 2.3a) is assumed to result from hormonal disturbance, but studies have failed to show a convincing hormonal abnormality in the majority of women. It has been shown that women who want treatment for their cyclical mastalgia have abnormal levels of anxiety, which fluctuate with their cycle. It is likely that cyclical mastalgia is an entirely normal phenomenon and that the real problem in women who continue to seek treatment after reassurance is anxiety.

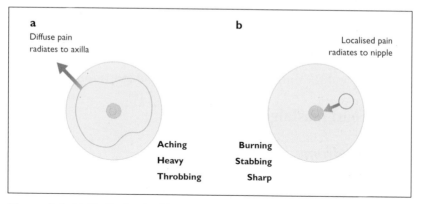

Figure 2.3. (a) Cyclical pain. (b) Non-cyclical pain: the features of pain caused by periductal mastitis.

Non-cyclical mastalgia

There are a number of non-cyclical mastalgia diagnoses, and pre- and post-menopausal women may experience symptoms. Careful clinical examination and history can establish the diagnosis. A diary chart of symptoms may also be helpful.

Duct ectasia and/or periductal mastitis (trigger spot pain)

Trigger spot pain has no regular pattern and random exacerbations may occur (occasionally during the premenstruum). It is often worse during cold weather. The site of the pain may be located precisely by the patient on each visit to the clinic. The sub areola, nipple and inner quadrant of the breast are the sites most commonly affected. The pain is often associated with a nipple discharge that is yellow or green in colour and the patient describes a burning or sharp pain.

Trauma

Pain caused by trauma may occur at the site of a previous surgical scar or previous injury. Pain has been reported at the site of a surgical incision biopsy that was followed by haematoma, or at the site of a previously drained abscess.

Breast cancer

Breast pain may be the presenting symptom for breast cancer (up to 10% cases). In these cases, pain is localized to the site of the tumour. In some cases a definite lump is palpable, in other cases there is a diffuse lumpiness, and for some patients no palpable lesion is found.

Non-breast mastalgia

Tietze syndrome

Tietze syndrome is not a true breast pain because the painful area, which can be established on careful examination, is the costochondral junction. The site of the pain is strongly localized, with only this area affected.

Lateral chest wall pain

Likewise, musculoskeletal pain may be experienced at the lateral chest wall. The pain is often described as an ache, or (less commonly) as a soreness, or as a drawing, throbbing sensation. The pain is intermittent in nature.

Cervical root syndrome

Nerve route pain from the cervical spine can be associated with pain in the upper outer part of the breast. It extends to the neck, shoulder and along the lateral aspect of the ipsilateral arm. It is often associated with limited movement of the cervical spine and paraesthesia in the affected arm. Radiographs of the affected area may show some changes associated with cervical spondylosis (Fig. 2.4).

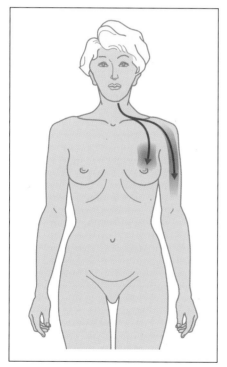

Figure 2.4. The distribution of pain from cervical spondylosis.

Miscellaneous or idiopathic

Pain in the breast may be the presenting symptom for a variety of conditions, including fibroadenoma (rare), pregnancy, depression, hiatus hernia, cholelithiasis, myocardial infarction and tuberculosis.

DISCHARGE

Discharge can be classified into three types – galactorrhoea, blood-related and opalescent.

Galactorrhoea

In galactorrhoea, the milky discharge is usually bilateral and from multiple ducts. It is common in late pregnancy and may persist for a long time after breast-feeding has stopped. The main causes are given in the box. Physiological galactorrhoea and galactorrhoea secondary to drug therapy do not require any treatment. Prolactinoma is a theoretical but extremely rare cause of galactorrhoea.

CAUSES OF GALACTORRHOEA

- Physiological

- Oral contraceptive pill

- Penothiazine therapy

- Thyroid disorders

- Prolactinoma

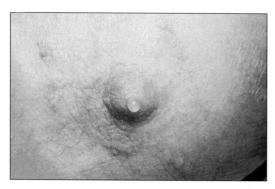

Figure 2.5. Clear discharge from a single duct of the nipple. This patient was found to have an intraduct carcinoma.

Blood-related discharge

Blood-related discharges may be clear and watery, but are usually serous (Fig. 2.5), serosanguinous or frank blood. The most common cause is an intraduct papilloma, which is benign and is not thought to have a malignant potential. About 5% are the result of intraduct carcinoma.

Opalescent discharge

Opalescent discharges are the most common types to present. The discharge can range in colour from yellow through green to brown and black. It may be unilateral or bilateral and frequently affects more than one duct in the breast. It results from duct ectasia and is benign.

DISTORTION

The most common distortion to present is nipple inversion, which may take two forms – horizontal and circumferential (Fig. 2.6). Horizontal retraction is likely to result from duct ectasia and/or periductal mastitis. Circumferential retraction is almost certainly caused by cancer.

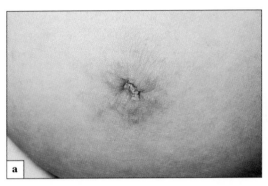

Figure 2.6. (a) Horizontal retraction. In this case there is crusting of the nipple, but this is not an invariable finding. (b) Circumferential retraction. In this case there is associated erythema of the skin. This is unusual, but signs other than the retraction are usually present.

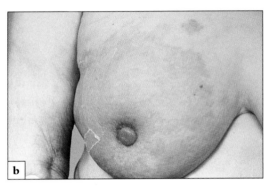

Rashes that affect the nipple

Paget's disease of the nipple

Paget's disease of the nipple (Fig. 2.7) is always associated with an underlying intraduct carcinoma. It is distinguished from other rashes that affect the nipple because it gives rise to actual destruction of the nipple. It is unilateral.

Eczema of the nipple

Eczema of the nipple usually occurs in patients with a history of eczema elsewhere. It is often bilateral, and there is no destruction of the nipple.

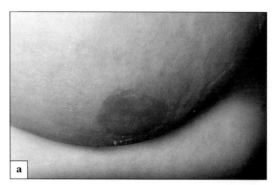

Figure 2.7. (a) Paget's disease of the nipple. (b) In the close up view, the destruction of the nipple can be clearly seen.

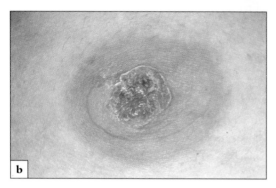

Scabies of the nipple

Scabies of the nipple is intensely itchy. It is usually associated with scabies elsewhere.

BREAST ABSCESS

Puerperal and lactational breast abscess

Breast abscess occurs in women who are breast-feeding. The usual portal of entry is a cracked nipple and the usual organism is *Staphylococcus aureus*.

Breast abscess secondary to duct ectasia and periductal mastitis

Breast abscesses are more commonly seen in women who are neither pregnant nor breast-feeding. The underlying pathology is duct ectasia with periductal mastitis, and the problem is more common in smokers. The exact mechanism by which smoking produces the problem is unknown. The organisms involved are usually anaerobes, although *S. aureus* may on occasion be implicated. If left untreated or treated inadequately, the abscess may result in the formation of a chronic *mammary duct fistula*, which may lead to recurrent episodes of infection.

CASE STUDIES

Case study 2.1

EF is a 28-year-old woman who attends for a regular check as she is on ethinyloestradiol with levonorgestrol (Microgynon). She mentions that for the past 3 months she has experienced a milky discharge from both breasts.

Discussion

SJL Provided there is no other abnormality on clinical examination, I would reassure her without any further investigations.

CT How confident can a GP be that the discharge is a result of the Pill?

SJL All the pathological causes of galactorrhoea are so rare that the Pill has to be regarded as the cause. I would be entirely confident in this case.

TG Can a milky discharge ever be an indication of underlying carcinoma?

SJL I have never heard of it. If a patient with galactorrhoea was found to have a breast cancer, I would regard it as coincidental.

TG Should the GP try changing from one Pill to another, or should it be stopped?

SJL There is no absolute indication for changing the Pill if the patient is otherwise happy with it and is content to put up with the discharge. If she wants to change, it might be worth trying a progesterone-only formulation, if that is compatible with her contraceptive needs. Progesterone-only Pills do not seem to give rise to galactorrhoea.

Case study 2.2

GH is a 45-year-old woman, who is married with two teenage children. For the past 6 months she has noticed a greenish-black discharge from her left breast. It is always present when she attempts to express it, but on several occasions has leaked out and stained her clothing.

Discussion

CT Is there any way of telling simply that this discharge is not altered blood?

SJL Yes; the Dipstix used to test for haematuria is just as effective in the detection of blood in a nipple discharge. A drop of the discharge applied to the appropriate square on the Dipstix gives the answer.

TG If a woman has a purulent discharge, is it likely to become a chronic problem?

SJL It is likely to become chronic, but it may not become a problem. If the discharge occurs only when it is expressed by the patient, simply advising the patient to refrain from expressing it may be all that is needed. (The management is discussed later – see Chapter 4.)

CT Is a woman who has a purulent discharge more at risk of developing a breast cancer in the future?

SJL The discharge does not in itself indicate an increased risk of breast cancer. Benign breast disease is only a risk factor for breast cancer when certain pathological changes are present. The usual cause of purulent discharge is duct ectasia, which is not associated with an increased risk of cancer.

Case study 2.3

JK is a 56-year-old woman who woke on the morning of her presentation with blood stains on her nightgown, apparently coming from her right nipple.

Discussion

TG Is a blood-stained discharge an early presentation of an intraduct carcinoma and if so does it have a better prognosis?

SJL Intraduct carcinoma is usually picked up at screening. If the tumour is near the nipple, it may present symptomatically with bloody discharge. The prognosis of treated *in situ* carcinoma is excellent whatever the method of detection. If it has not become invasive, then adequate local treatment is curative.

CT Is there any cause for a blood-stained discharge other than intraduct papilloma or intraduct carcinoma? I know someone who had a blood-stained discharge during pregnancy and was reassured.

SJL Blood-stained discharge may occur during late pregnancy or early puerperium and is described well in the older textbooks. It is thought to be related to the dilatation of the blood vessels that surround the ducts and is not of any pathological significance. It is not a contraindication to breast-feeding.

Case study 2.4

MN is 70-year-old woman who presents because she noticed that her nipple has become indrawn over the past 3 months. She has some discomfort in the breast and occasionally finds white crusting on the nipple. There is no palpable mass.

Discussion

TG As MN doesn't have a palpable lump, is it less likely that her symptoms are the result of a carcinoma?

SJL If there is no palpable lump and the indrawing is of the horizontal slit type, it is very unlikely that she has a carcinoma.

CT If she had a discharge in addition to her indrawn nipple would she be more likely to have a carcinoma?

SJL The diagnosis depends on the nature of the discharge. Purulent discharge and a horizontal slit nipple are both the result of duct ectasia and/or periductal mastitis, and carcinoma is unlikely. A blood stained discharge suggests the possibility of an underlying cancer, as it would even if the nipple were not indrawn.

Case study 2.5

OP is 51 years old, nulliparous and has been using oestradiol only (Estraderm) for 2 years. She presents complaining of a lump in her right breast.

Discussion

CT Is her nulliparity significant?

SJL As she is nulliparous, she has a higher risk of breast cancer. However, this does not really influence our thinking in coming to a diagnosis. Since breast cancer is so common, the reduction in risk in a parous woman does not allow us to discount the possibility of breast cancer when she presents with a lump.

TG Does the fact that she has been on HRT for 2 years increase her risk of breast cancer?

SJL The meta-analysis of HRT studies now shows fairly clearly that there is a small increase in the risk of developing breast cancer in women who are on HRT for 5–10 years. At 5 years the relative risk is 1.023. The mortality from breast cancer is not increased. At 2 years there is no detectable increase in risk.

TG Are benign breast lumps more common in women who take HRT?

SJL All forms of benign breast disease are more common in women taking HRT.

Case study 2.6

RS (34 years of age) comes to the surgery to tell you that her 45-year-old sister has been diagnosed as having breast cancer. She wants to know whether she can have screening and whether there is any treatment she can take.

Discussion

CT Does RS have an increased risk of developing breast cancer and is it dependent on whether her sister was pre- or post-menopausal at the time of diagnosis?

SJL This is not entirely straightforward. To answer the easy part first, the data with regard to family history are related to age not menopausal status, so the sister's menopausal status is irrelevant to our calculations. An individual is regarded as being at high risk of breast cancer if one first-degree relative under 40 or two first-degree relatives under 50 years of age have breast cancer. A first-degree relative with bilateral breast cancer is also a marker of high risk. When only one 45-year-old member of the family is affected the increase in risk is less. We would regard RS as being at medium risk, with a relative risk of around 1.5. An additional history of prostate cancer in male members of the family would move her into the high-risk category.

CT Should RS have screening and if so what should that consist of?

SJL Once again, this is a complex question. There is no firm evidence that screening women with a family history of cancer effectively reduces mortality from breast cancer. Remember, it is not enough to show that screening can detect the disease. Before it can be universally recommended, it has to be shown that it reduces mortality from the disease. Moving away from the theoretical into the realm of practical clinical management, it may be necessary to offer screening to RS for psychological support. This should be annual mammography as she is 34 years old; if screening is to make an impact on those under 50, it probably has to be carried out annually.

TG Does tamoxifen taken prophylactically reduce some women's risk of developing breast cancer and if so which women? What sort of problems could this cause in the long term?

SJL The evidence at present is unclear. The American trial of prophylactic tamoxifen was terminated early because they thought they had convincing proof that it was effective. Two European studies have failed to show any benefit. There is much discussion over this discrepancy and the jury is still out. The ISIS trial is still ongoing and perhaps its results will clarify matters. The main worry long term is the development of endometrial cancer.

CHAPTER SUMMARY

- There are four main symptoms of breast disease – lump, pain, discharge and distortion.
- Lumpiness of the breast should be distinguished from a true lump. Lumpiness does not need to be investigated, but a lump should be fully investigated. Deciding between the two is very difficult at times.
- Cyclical mastalgia is related to hormonal changes. It does not need extensive investigation.
- Non-cyclical mastalgia has a variety of causes. If it presents as a new symptom investigation is warranted.
- Galactorrhoea is usually physiological or drug-induced; coloured discharges are harmless; clear, serous or bloodstained discharges may arise from intraduct carcinoma and should be investigated.
- Long-standing abnormalities of the nipple are the result of benign conditions. Recent changes are probably caused by benign disease, but may need to be investigated.
- Breast abscesses and inflammatory conditions are often caused by anaerobic organisms and should be treated with antibiotics that are effective against anaerobes.

chapter 3

The diagnosis of breast disease

As a result of the high level of awareness of breast disease generated by health promotion campaigns and by the media, a large number of women are presenting to their GP with breast symptoms. While some women find these symptoms because they practise regular breast self-examination (BSE) and some symptoms are found at well women clinics, the majority are found by chance.

BREAST SELF-EXAMINATION AND ROUTINE CLINICAL EXAMINATION

The early detection of breast cancer results in an improvement in outcome. It seems obvious that if women are encouraged to carry out regular BSE, breast cancers will be detected at an earlier stage. Some of the literature suggests that this is indeed the case. When breast cancers are classified into those detected by routine BSE and those detected by chance, those detected by BSE are smaller and the chance that they have metastasized into the axilla is lower. However, studies of teaching BSE to populations have not shown any improvement in the stage at which breast cancer presents. This may be related to poor compliance with BSE in the trial population. The women who do consistently practice BSE tend to be in the younger age group in whom the risk of breast cancer is low. The group that is at risk tends not to practice BSE.

There are concerns that the inappropriate emphasis on BSE in the younger women leads to an increase in the number of benign lumps that are presented. This leads to an increase in the number of investigations, including open biopsies, and also gives rise to needless anxiety in the women. The response in the UK has been to move away from the promotion of regular BSE to the encouragement of breast awareness. Women are discouraged from carrying out regular BSE, but are encouraged to report any changes in the breast as soon as they are detected. The media give frequent high-profile coverage to breast disease, which certainly encourages breast awareness and has resulted in an increased number of women presenting with breast symptoms.

The role of opportunistic clinical examination of the breast as a screening tool is also unclear. In the past it was routine practice to examine women's breasts when they attend for cervical smear or prescription of the contraceptive pill or HRT. This was frequently performed by specialist nurses. The Chief Medical Officer and Chief Nursing Officer in the UK Department of Health have issued a joint letter that discourages this practice, since lesions may be missed and false reassurance be given to the woman. As there is clear evidence from the literature that trained nurses are effective in detecting breast cancer by clinical examination, there is an argument that training should be extended to nurses who are involved in well women clinics, rather than stopping opportunistic screening.

MANAGING THE WOMAN WITH BREAST SYMPTOMS

Whatever the mode of detection of the breast symptoms, the woman with those symptoms is likely to be anxious. Recent high-profile cases of 'missed diagnosis' make it difficult to reassure women without giving them a thorough investigation. On the other hand, if every woman with breast symptoms were to be investigated, the system would break down under the strain.

A routine needs to be introduced that will allow vetting of women so that those who are most likely to have serious disease can be dealt with speedily. Guidelines have been published by the National Health Service Breast Screening Programme (NHSBSP) and disseminated to GPs by the Royal College of General Practitioners (RCGP). Figures 3.1–3.4 are adapted from those guidelines.

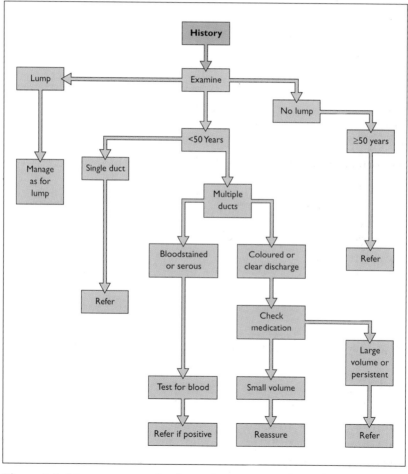

Figure 3.1. Management routine for vetting women with nipple discharge.

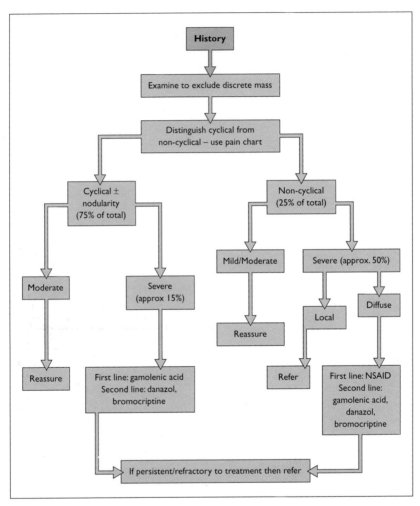

Figure 3.2. Management routine for vetting women with breast pain.

Once the patient arrives in the Breast Unit, the full diagnostic process is instituted. The exact diagnostic pathway depends on the patient's age and symptoms, but is likely to involve some form of the triple assessment that comprises clinical examination, imaging and tissue diagnosis. Up to 50% of women who attend the Breast Unit are found to have no abnormality. Presumably, the symptoms are self-limiting and resolve before the

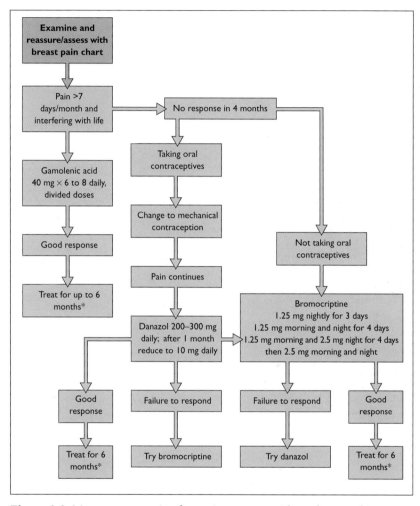

Figure 3.3. Management routine for vetting women with moderate and/or severe cyclical mastalgia. Mild mastalgia requires examination and reassurance. * After 6 months treatment should be stopped. In only half of patients will breast pains recur, and some of these will not need further treatment because pain is milder. Severe recurrences can be treated with a further course of previously successful treatment.

patient reaches the specialist. In such cases the clinician may decide not to pursue further investigations, especially so for younger patients.

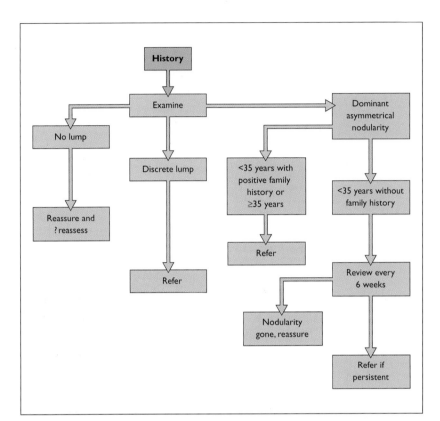

Figure 3.4. Management routine for vetting women with a breast lump.

Clinical examination

Clinical examination remains an important component of the diagnostic process and in expert hands is both sensitive and specific. Concerns that examination by non-experts may give rise to a false sense of security in women with actual disorders, who are therefore inappropriately reassured, are best answered by increasing the number of practitioners with the requisite skills. There is clear evidence from the literature that trained nurses are effective at detecting breast disease by clinical examination.

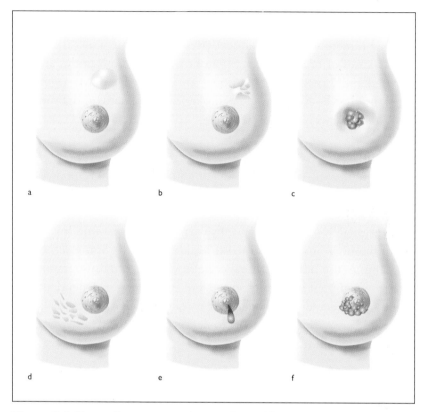

Figure 3.5. Signs of breast cancer that may be visible on inspection. (a) Lump; (b) dimpling; (c) recent nipple inversion; (d) peau d'orange; (e) serous or blood stained discharge; (f) Paget's disease of nipple. Lumps are usually detected by palpation. Discharge may be visible only when attempt is made to express it.

A number of different approaches may be made to clinical examination. It does not matter which approach is used, as long as the examination is carried out systematically. Inspection is important and the important element in inspection is comparison between the two sides. Palpation is carried out using the flat of the fingers, and all the quadrants of the breast must be covered. Attention should be paid to the area behind the nipple and discharge should be looked for routinely (Fig. 3.5).

Examination of the axilla should always be undertaken, although it must be remembered that clinical assessment of the axilla is inaccurate. In cases of breast cancer, 50% of involved lymph nodes are not palpated and 25% of palpable nodes are not involved. Management decisions must be based on the pathological node status as determined by histological examination.

Imaging

Two main imaging modalities – mammography and ultrasonography – are routinely used. In mammography the breast is compressed in the lateral oblique or craniocaudal planes while a radiograph is taken using conventional X-rays (Fig. 3.6). In carrying out mammography on symptomatic women it is usual to use both views. Some screening programmes use only the lateral oblique view. In ultrasonography the breast is examined using ultrasound, but it is operator dependent and is not a good screening modality. It is useful to characterize palpable masses and areas of nodularity or to define further the nature of masses detected by mammography.

Mammography

In women over 40 years old, mammography is very sensitive in detecting abnormalities. It is less effective in younger women, as the breast tissue in younger women is radiographically dense (Fig. 3.7). In older women, HRT can increase the radiographic density of the breast and may reduce the effectiveness of mammographic screening.

When mammograms are being read a comparison is made between the breasts. Three major types of abnormality are looked for – microcalcifications, masses and stromal deformities. Asymmetric density may or may not be significant, but certainly warrants further imaging.

Microcalcification

Microcalcification can occur in benign breast disease or be associated with breast cancer, particularly ductal carcinoma *in situ*. The classic

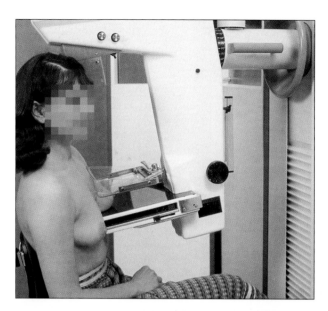

Figure 3.6.
A woman undergoing mammography. Note the breast is compressed by the mammogram machine. This may be uncomfortable but is not usually painful.

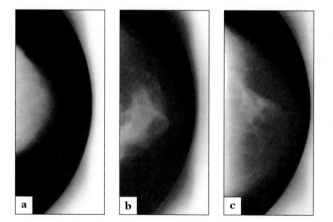

Figure 3.7. A comparison of mammograms in patients of different ages.
(a) Mammogram taken of a 35-year-old woman. Note the uniform density of the image, which may make it difficult to see small lesions. (b) As the patient ages, the radiographic density of the breast decreases. In anatomical terms, it is not clear why this occurs. HRT can increase the radiographic density of the breast.
(c) Mammogram taken of an older woman with larger breasts. Most of the breast tissue is replaced by fat. Small lesions are readily visible in this sort of breast.

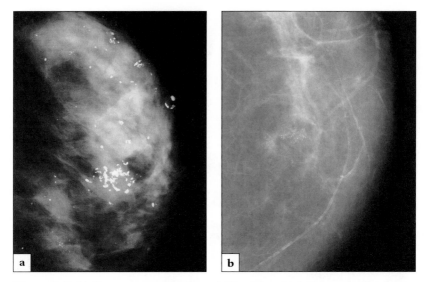

Figure 3.8. (a) Coarse scattered microcalcification, which is typical of benign disease. Fine needle aspiration was reported as benign and no biopsy was performed. (b) A tight cluster of irregular microcalcification. This proved on biopsy to be an area of ductal carcinoma *in situ*.

appearances of benign microcalcification (Fig. 3.8a) and malignant calcification (Fig. 3.8b) are very different, but in practice it may be impossible to decide whether the appearances are the result of carcinoma. The microcalcification is then said to be indeterminate and further investigations must be carried out.

Masses

Benign masses, such as cysts and fibroadenomas, are classically regular in shape with a well-defined outline (Fig. 3.9). Fibroadenomas may be lobulated and in older women often contain coarse calcification as a result of involution. Malignant masses may have an irregular outline and are often spiculated (Fig. 3.10). Any mass visible on mammography should be examined with ultrasound to help define its nature as some forms of cancer, such as medullary carcinoma, may look very like a fibroadenoma.

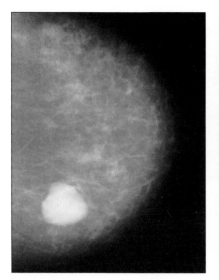

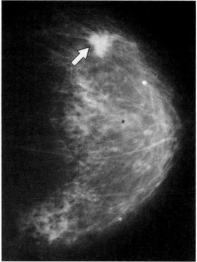

Figure 3.9. A typical fibroadenoma. The lesion is dense and the edge is well delineated. There is no evidence of involution in this particular lesion.

Figure 3.10. A typical carcinoma (arrow). Note the irregular margin and the associated spiculation.

Stromal deformities

Most stromal deformities are so-called radial scars, which are entirely benign. However, similar mammographic appearances can be seen with small tubular carcinomas.

Further investigations

When abnormalities are found on mammography, it may be helpful to carry out further views with compression and magnification of the area. This may resolve the question entirely; for example, an apparently asymmetric density may be found to result from overlapping shadows of normal glandular structures, or an apparent stromal deformity may disappear.

Ultrasound is very helpful in the diagnosis of masses. Some are found to be simple cysts (Fig. 3.11), which are easily diagnosed on ultrasound. Unless they are symptomatic they can be left alone without further

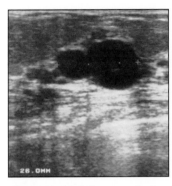 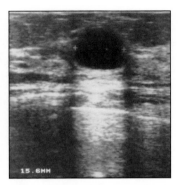

Figure 3.11. Ultrasound of typical cyst. The margin is well defined. There are no echoes within the lesion and there is enhancement (the bright band) behind the lesion.

investigation or treatment. Solid masses may have characteristic appearances that suggest fibroadenoma or carcinoma (Fig. 3.12), but confirmation of the diagnosis is usually sought by either aspiration cytology or needle biopsy.

Ultrasound also helps in deciding whether a palpable lesion is a discrete mass or is an area of nodularity resulting from benign breast change or prominent glandular tissue.

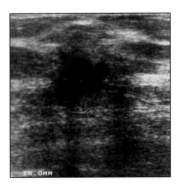 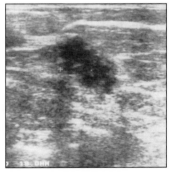

Figure 3.12. Ultrasound of typical carcinoma. The edges of the lesion are irregular. There is a mixed pattern of echoes within the lesion. Some 'acoustic shadowing' is seen.

Fine-needle aspiration cytology

When suction from a standard 10 or 20 ml syringe is applied to a 21 or 23FG needle that is passed backward and forward through an area of breast tissue, sufficient material is drawn into the needle to allow a diagnosis to be made by an expert cytologist. Ideally, for a successful aspirate for cytology, no material should appear in the syringe. The contents of the needle are expelled onto a series of microscope slides and spread as a smear. The material on the slide can be fixed by rapid air-drying or by immersion in alcohol, depending on the preference of the cytopathologist who is to report them. Air-dried slides are stained with haematoxylin and eosin. Alcohol-fixed slides are stained with Papinicolaou's stain. Results may be reported immediately or certainly within 24 hours.

Even in expert hands insufficient cellular material for diagnosis is obtained in up to 20% of cases. By convention, this outcome is designated C_1 – inadequate for diagnosis. The other categories are:

- C_2 – definitely benign
- C_3 – suspicious, but probably benign
- C_4 – suspicious, probably malignant
- C_5 – definitely malignant.

The C_2 category may simply be reported as adequate and benign when no specific features are present, but could be reported as showing specific features of fibroadenoma, fibrocystic change or cyst.

Wide-bore needle biopsy

A variety of wide-bore needles can be used to obtain a core of tissue for formal histological diagnosis. Processing and reporting take longer than for fine-needle aspiration cytology, but it is possible to distinguish between *in situ* and invasive carcinoma, which is not possible with cytology. The reported categories are analogous to those for cytology, although it is less likely that an inadequate specimen will be obtained.

Both forms of tissue diagnosis are subject to sampling error and in some centres a second biopsy is carried out after an interval to confirm the report. In other centres, the biopsy is repeated only if the result does not match the findings of imaging and clinical examination.

The triple assessment approach

When the investigations have been completed, the clinician must make a decision based on the findings. If all of the modalities (including clinical examination) suggest that the lesion is benign, the patient can be reassured that there is no cause for concern. If all modalities are consistent with malignancy, the patient can be told that she has cancer and treatment plans can be discussed.

When there is a discrepancy between the modalities, further biopsy must be carried out. When any modality suggests malignancy, formal excision biopsy must be performed even if the other modalities suggest that the lesion is benign. If this rule is adhered to, it is safe not to biopsy every breast lump that presents. It is almost inevitable that the diagnosis of some cancers is delayed because all the indications on the triple assessment suggest that the lump is benign and a judgement is taken that the lump does not need to be excised. Even when there is a policy of excising all breast lumps a judgement has to be made as to what constitutes a lump that needs biopsy. Errors of judgement lead to a delay in diagnosis whatever the approach adopted. It is important to appreciate this and not to apportion blame when a breast cancer is missed, providing all the necessary measures to ensure a diagnosis have been undertaken.

GIVING THE PATIENT THE DIAGNOSIS

There are two different approaches to giving the patient the diagnosis. In some units the patient is told on the day of first attending the unit. Other units prefer to bring the patients back several days later to tell them the diagnosis. The protagonists of each view claim that their approach is better for the patients' psychological well-being, but no formal comparison of the two approaches has yet been made. When the diagnosis turns out to be benign there is no obvious benefit in making the patient wait; when the diagnosis turns out to be cancer a staged breaking of the news may make it easier to accept. On the other hand, most women who attend with a breast lump fear the worst and a diagnosis of cancer does not come as a shock to them.

Ideally, the patient should be accompanied by a friend or relative when the diagnosis is discussed. It is common practice now for the doctor to be accompanied by a breast-care nurse during this phase of the consultation. Once the diagnosis has been given and understood, the treatment options can be discussed.

CHAPTER SUMMARY

- Women should be encouraged to be breast aware and taught the important signs of breast cancer.
- Referral to a specialist unit should be based on the NHSBSP guidelines disseminated by the RCGP.
- Diagnosis in the Breast Unit is based on the triple assessment, with clinical examination, imaging and tissue diagnosis (usually by fine-needle aspiration cytology).
- Up to 50% of women who present to the Breast Unit have no abnormality detected. If this is the case it may be decided, especially in younger women, not to pursue all the investigations.
- If there is any remaining doubt after the triple assessment, the patient should undergo open biopsy.
- The diagnostic process should be completed as expeditiously as possible to minimize the patient's anxiety.

chapter 4

The management of benign breast disease

The majority of who women present with breast symptoms do not have breast cancer. Of women who attend a breast clinic, 50% are found to have entirely normal breasts on examination and investigation. A further 40% have benign disease. One of the most important objectives in the management of these patients is reassurance that there is no evidence of malignancy. Women with breast symptoms are commonly afraid that they have cancer.

DIAGNOSIS

A careful diagnostic approach, including *triple assessment* where appropriate, is in itself the first stage toward reassuring the patient. As far as possible, a firm diagnosis should be reached during the first episode. While it is occasionally necessary to review a patient after an interval to be sure of the diagnosis, there is little justification for regular follow-up of a patient with benign disease.

While some patients who report breast symptoms are relieved merely by being told they do not have cancer, other women seek a full explanation of the cause of their symptoms and others remain sufficiently troubled by their symptoms to request an appropriate treatment.

BENIGN BREAST CHANGE (Fig. 4.1)

Benign breast change usually presents as diffuse nodularity or thickening. If there is no associated pain the woman does not usually need treatment beyond the reassurance of a diagnosis. The decision that must be made is whether to investigate the patient further or to reassure her on the basis of clinical examination. As a result of the high level of anxiety that breast disease engenders the tendency is to overinvestigate, even in specialist breast clinics.

BREAST CYST (Fig. 4.1)

When a discrete lump is present, needle aspiration is indicated. If this is the patient's first presentation, this should be carried out in the

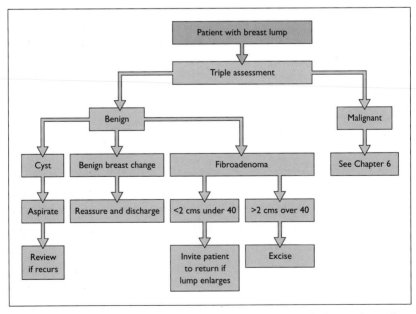

Figure 4.1. Management routine for patient presenting with discrete breast lump.

specialist clinic as part of the triple assessment. If the lump is a cyst, it is aspirated to extinction. Provided no residual lump remains and the fluid is not bloodstained, cytology is not necessary. It is traditional, but probably unnecessary, to re-examine the patient after 4–6 weeks to make sure that the cyst has not recurred. Recurrence is infrequent and the patient would usually return anyway if she finds that the lump has recurred.

If a patient is known to have recurring cysts and presents with another lump, it is sensible for the GP to carry out the needle aspiration to save the patient a trip to the clinic. Once again, the rules apply that if there is no residual lump and the fluid is not bloodstained no further action is required. If there is a residual lump this must be fully investigated by triple assessment.

A few patients have cysts that recur so frequently that the patient wants some form of therapy to stop them developing. The most useful therapy in these circumstances is danazol 100 mg twice a day, which should be taken for at least 6 months. Patients with recurrent cysts do have a higher-than-normal risk of developing breast cancer, so even if the patient is known to have recurrent cysts, every new lump must be subjected to aspiration or ultrasound examination.

FIBROADENOMA (Fig. 4.1)

In women under 40 years of age, small (<2 cm) fibroadenomas that have been confirmed on triple assessment do not need to be removed. Some surgeons recommend regular follow-up of these patients in case the lump begins to enlarge. Most patients can be relied upon to monitor their own lump with instructions to report back if it appears to change.

When the lump is over 2 cm or the woman is over 40 years of age, the tendency is to recommend excision of the lump even when it is shown to be a fibroadenoma. This is probably another example of over-caution, but is the accepted practice.

BREAST PAIN (Fig. 4.2)

One of the most common presenting problems is breast pain. As described in Chapter 2, breast pain may be classified as cyclical, non-cyclical and non-breast. A careful history and examination usually distinguishes these. When the nature and periodicity of the pain is unclear, it is helpful to ask the patient to record a pain diary for several months. Pain that is essentially cyclical in its aetiology can become continuous as it becomes more severe. Patients with breast pain do not usually have any palpable lump and, if the pain is clearly cyclical, no further investigation is needed beyond simple breast examination. If the pain is of recent onset and non-cyclical or if there is an associated lump, the patient should be referred for *triple assessment*.

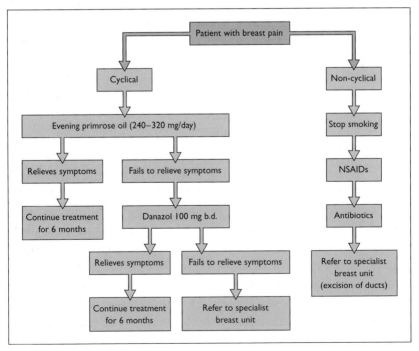

Figure 4.2. Management routine for patient presenting with breast pain.

Cyclical mastalgia

Women with mild-to-moderate symptoms are probably reassured by exclusion of malignancy and an explanation of their symptoms. Those women who tend to seek treatment are those with more persistent pain that is present for more than 1 week in each menstrual cycle. The pain tends to be severe in intensity so that it interferes with their lifestyle and normal activities. By the time the patients seek treatment the pain has usually persisted for several months. Some of these women may be suffering from a clinical anxiety state and others may be depressed. Worsening of their mood is associated with the luteal phase of the menstrual cycle.

If the patient continues to want treatment after she has been reassured that no serious disease is present, gamolenic acid (evening primrose oil, 240–320 mg per day in divided doses) is recommended as the first line. The patient should be warned that no effect may be noticed for 2–3 months. Treatment should continue for a minimum of 3 months before trying a second line of treatment.

For those women satisfied with the response (as indicated by improved recording on their pain chart) treatment should continue until a 6-month course has been completed. At this stage the treatment should be stopped, because for many women a single course of treatment resolves their symptoms. Some women remain free of symptoms, while others have a recurrence of symptoms but do not seek further treatment as the symptoms do not become severe. A number of women require a further course of treatment because the pain returns at the same level as previously.

For those patients who fail to respond to first-line treatment a hormonal manipulation should prove more successful.

If the patient is on the oral contraceptive, breast symptoms may be relieved by a change of oral contraceptive. If this fails, it may help to stop the oral contraceptive and use a mechanical method.

If the patient is not taking oral contraceptives, danazol 200–300 mg daily for 1 month, reducing to 100 mg daily, will probably be successful. The patient should be warned of the possible side effects; the most common of these is nausea, but the one that concerns most women is weight gain. Other side effects include acne and hirsutism. The incidence of troublesome side effects is about 10%. If treatment is successful it should be continued for 6 months, and if symptoms recur a further course can be prescribed.

Patients who do not respond to danazol are difficult to manage and should probably be referred to a specialist breast unit. A number of options are available.

Bromocriptine may be effective, but its usefulness is limited by the incidence of side effects. It should be administered in incremental doses (to minimize side effects) – 1.25 mg for 3 days; 1.25 mg twice daily for 4 days; 1.25 mg in the morning and 2.5 mg in the afternoon for 4 days; and finally 2.5 mg twice daily.

Tamoxifen and goserelin have been shown in clinical trials to be effective in relieving cyclical mastalgia, but these drugs are not licensed for this purpose. The specialist may decide to use them on a named-patient basis in cases that are resistant to other therapies.

Diuretic therapy, exclusion diets and diet supplements with vitamins B_1, B_6 and E have all been recommended at various times, but their benefit is not proved and they should not be prescribed. Advice such as wearing a better-fitting bra and restricting fluid intake during the luteal phase of the cycle is also ineffective.

Non-cyclical breast pain

Non-cyclical breast pain is difficult to treat. The underlying problem is usually inflammatory and can sometimes respond to a non-steroidal anti-inflammatory drug. The inflammation is often caused by anaerobic organisms. Treatment with appropriate antibiotics, such as metronidazole or co-amoxiclav, may relieve the symptoms in the short term, but recurrence is common once the antibiotics are stopped. It is undesirable for the patient to remain on antibiotics for long periods and the use of antibiotics should be reserved for particular episodes when the pain is very severe.

Smoking exacerbates the inflammatory process and patients who are smokers should be told that their symptoms are unlikely to respond to treatment. Often cessation of smoking in itself leads to the disappearance of the pain.

In resistant cases it is occasionally necessary to excise the central duct system within the breast. The patient should understand before consenting to the operation that success in relieving the pain cannot be guaranteed.

Where pain is localized to a single tender area within the breast (trigger spot), some women benefit from an injection of local anaesthetic and corticosteroid. Rarely is surgical excision of the tender spot appropriate, because some women develop pain at the site of previous breast surgery.

Gamolenic acid (240–320 mg per day, in divided doses) can be prescribed, but is likely to be less effective than it is in cyclical mastalgia.

Non-breast pain

Pain that is localized to the costochondral junction (Tietze syndrome) or other part of the chest wall and is persistent in nature can be treated effectively by infiltration with local anaesthetic and corticosteroid injection (2 ml, 1% lignocaine [4% lidocaine] with 40 mg methyl-prednisolone in 1 ml). This should result in the complete disappearance of the pain for a period of time. Some women may require a repeat injection 2–3 months later.

Other pains that are not breast in origin are treated most effectively once the cause of the symptoms has been established and the diagnosis confirmed. For example, if the pain is cardiac or gastric in nature, then appropriate management and symptom relief should relieve the symptoms.

NIPPLE DISCHARGE

The treatment of galactorrhoea is to treat the underlying cause. When this is drug-induced, and continued treatment with the drug is necessary or desirable, the patient can be reassured that the discharge is of no importance. If the drug concerned is the contraceptive pill, a change to a different pill may result in disappearance of the symptom. However, an underlying hormonal disorder requires referral to an endocrinologist.

The multi-coloured, multi-duct discharge of duct ectasia does not require treatment, except for symptomatic relief. If the discharge occurs only when the patient expresses it, she should be discouraged from doing so. If it occurs spontaneously, especially if it occurs at inconvenient times, she should be instructed to express it completely in the bath or shower.

Occasionally, the discharge is so troublesome that surgical removal of the milk ducts is necessary. This procedure should not be undertaken lightly as the nipple will be rendered numb, which can in itself be distressing.

When the discharge is serous or bloodstained and from a single duct, a microdochectomy (removal of a single duct) must be performed to establish the diagnosis. Intraduct carcinoma cannot be excluded reliably by any other means. If an intraduct papilloma is found no further treatment is needed. Any cancer detected must receive treatment on its merits.

NIPPLE INVERSION OR RETRACTION

Nipple inversion does not require treatment. In young women who are concerned about the cosmetic appearance, a relatively minor surgical procedure can be undertaken to evert the nipple. The patient should be warned about altered sensation in the nipple and problems with lactation should she become pregnant.

BREAST ABSCESS

Outside of the puerperium, breast abscesses are usually associated with duct ectasia and infection with anaerobic organisms. The antibiotics of choice are those that are active against anaerobes, of which metronidazole and co-amoxiclav are the drugs of choice. If treatment is started in the cellulitic phase, abscess formation may be prevented. Once pus has formed the abscess should be aspirated before starting the antibiotics. If this is ineffective, the abscess will have to be formally drained under anaesthetic. It can be closed primarily under antibiotic cover or can be packed and allowed to granulate. Primary closure is preferable.

MAMMARY DUCT FISTULA

A mammary duct fistula does not heal spontaneously. It must be treated surgically by laying open, or preferably by excision.

NIPPLE ECZEMA

Eczema of the nipple can be treated as eczema anywhere else. Mild corticosteroid creams are usually effective.

CHAPTER SUMMARY

- The most important factor in managing benign breast disease is to establish a firm diagnosis as expeditiously as possible.
- Benign breast lumps do not need to be removed provided the diagnosis is soundly based on the triple assessment process.
- If patients can be reassured, it may not be necessary to treat breast pain.
- Cyclical breast pain is hormonal in origin and is responsive to a variety of treatments.
- Non-cyclical breast pain is usually inflammatory in origin and is often exacerbated by smoking.
- Patients with nipple discharge can be reassured that their condition is benign, unless the discharge is serous or bloodstained. If this is the case the patient should be investigated further.

chapter 5

The principles of treatment modalities

The treatment of breast cancer can appear confusing, particularly as best practice seems to change with bewildering frequency. To make some sense of the confusion, it is necessary to have a basic understanding of the principles that underlie the various treatment modalities and their utilization.

PRINCIPLES OF THE MANAGEMENT OF EARLY CANCER

The two principle goals in the management of early breast cancer are the long-term control of local disease and the prevention of distant disease. These two are inter-related, as the development of local recurrence may be associated with the subsequent development of metastases. Traditional approaches to breast cancer are based on the assumption that the disease spreads centrifugally, starting in the breast, then extending to the lymph nodes before finally being carried by the bloodstream to distant organs. On this basis, it seemed logical that larger and larger local operations would improve the outcome, but this did not prove to be the case. A revised concept of breast cancer was adopted that postulated systemic spread of the disease at an early stage in the development of the tumour, so that by the time the patient presents with a lump, metastases have already occurred. These are microscopic in the majority of cases and are not detectable by current methods of investigation. Clearly, no local treatment, however radical, will cure the patient if there are micro-metastases. For this reason, the concept of adjuvant treatment was introduced in the late 1960s and has become accepted as the standard management.

SURGERY

The major role of surgery (Fig. 5.1) is to give local control of the disease. The extent of surgery necessary to achieve this depends on the nature, location and size of the tumour and on the use of other treatment modalities. A secondary role of surgery at present is to help define disease extent by removal of axillary lymph nodes.

Wide local excision

Wide local excision is the removal of the tumour along with a margin of normal tissue. Surgeons vary as to the size of margin that they take. The outcome of this approach depends on the completeness of the excision and the biology of the tumour. Certain features of the tumour indicate an increased risk of local recurrence (Table 5.1).

It may not be advisable to carry out wide local excision if the lump is large in relation to the breast. The ensuing deformity might be cosmetically worse than that from a mastectomy with reconstruction.

When the lesion is directly behind the nipple, the wide local excision may be modified to include removing the nipple. It is then referred to as a central excision, but is otherwise no different than a wide local excision.

Mastectomy

Several approaches can be taken to mastectomy. The most common is a total mastectomy in which the breast is removed along with an ellipse of skin that includes the nipple. In the past this was often called a simple mastectomy to distinguish it from a radical mastectomy in

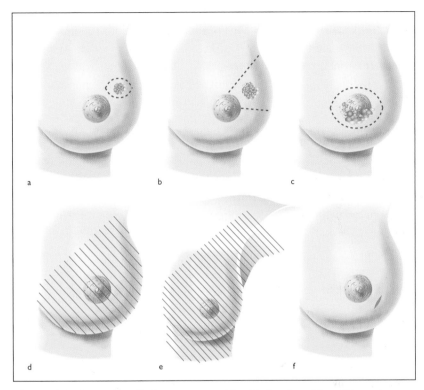

Figure 5.1. Operations for breast cancer: (a) wide local excision; (b) quadrant-ectomy; (c) central excision (removing nipple); (d) total mastectomy; (e) radical mastectomy (rarely performed now); (f) incision biopsy of inoperable cancer (largely replaced by needle biopsy). Axillary procedures may or may not be carried out with any of the above breast procedures except radical mastectomy, which always includes an axillary clearance.

which the breast was removed along with the axillary lymph nodes and the pectoral muscles. Note that the difference between a radical mastectomy and a total (or simple) mastectomy lies in what is removed with the breast, not in the amount of breast tissue removed. In 1948, David Patey showed that a complete clearance of the axillary nodes could be achieved without removing the pectoral muscles, and the modified radical mastectomy gradually replaced the radical

Table 5.1. Features of the tumour that indicate an increased risk of local recurrence after breast conservation.

Feature	Description
Extensive ductal carcinoma *in situ*	The presence of ductal carcinoma *in situ* (non-invasive) of more than 25% of the diameter of the invasive carcinoma
Involved excision margins	Histological evidence that the surgeon has cut through tumour in excising the lump
Presence of vascular and/or lymphatic invasion	Histological evidence of tumour within epithelial-lined structures in the breast; these are either blood vessels or lymphatics
Grade 3 tumour	This is a poorly differentiated tumour – premenopausal women with Grade 3 tumours have a higher risk of recurrence

mastectomy as the operation of choice. To avoid misunderstanding as to what is being removed, this is often referred to now as total mastectomy and axillary clearance.

Under some circumstances a subcutaneous mastectomy is performed. The nipple is preserved along with all of the skin, and a silicone implant may be inserted to restore the breast volume. There are two problems with this procedure. First, it is not possible to guarantee that all the breast tissue has been removed. When the indication for the operation is malignancy or the future risk of malignancy, the procedure may not be effective. Second, the cosmetic effect is often very poor. If the prosthesis is placed deep to the pectoralis major, the skin may become wrinkled and adhere to the muscle. If it is placed between the skin and the muscle to avoid the wrinkling, the incidence of capsular contraction (both unsightly and uncomfortable) is high.

Axillary procedures

The management of the axilla is one of the more controversial aspects in breast surgery. A number of procedures are performed.

Axillary sampling involves identifying four nodes and removing them. Proponents of this approach claim that it stages the axilla accurately and has a low incidence of morbidity. If nodes are found to be involved, radiotherapy is given to the axilla. It is difficult to identify the anatomical level from which the nodes have been removed.

In contrast, axillary clearance involves an anatomical dissection of the axilla and removal of clearly defined groups of nodes. The axilla is divided into notional levels by the pectoralis minor (Fig. 5.2):

- Nodes up to the lateral border of pectoralis minor lie in Level 1.
- Nodes deep to pectoralis minor lie in Level 2.
- Nodes medial to the medial border of pectoralis minor lie in Level 3.

Axillary clearances may be to any of the three levels. A properly conducted axillary clearance strips the fascia from the walls of the axilla, while preserving the nerves if possible. No lymph nodes should remain in the cleared area, but the more radical the clearance the greater the likelihood of lymphoedema developing – with a Level 3 clearance the chance of significant lymphoedema is 10%. On the other hand, if nodal involvement is found on a Level 1 clearance, it is prudent to treat the remaining nodal areas with radiotherapy, a procedure which has an incidence of lymphoedema similar to that of a Level 3 clearance.

Breast reconstruction

Breast reconstruction after mastectomy is not a new concept. When first introduced in the 1960s, it was thought that it could be carried out only after the patient had been disease free for at least 2 years. Studies of immediate reconstruction have shown no disadvantage to the patient, in terms of survival and recurrence, in carrying out the reconstruction immediately. There may be psychological benefit in doing so. A number of methods are available, described below.

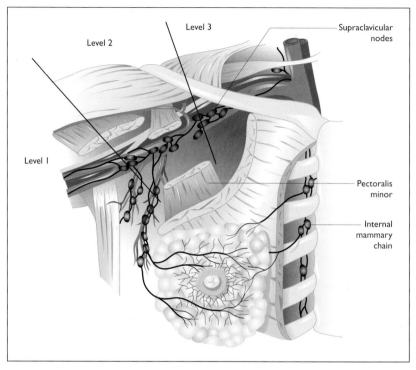

Figure 5.2. The lymph node groups that drain the breast. Note that the axillary nodes and supraclavicular nodes are in continuity with one another. The divisions between them are descriptive and artificial, not functional.

Tissue expanders and implants

The simplest technique for reconstruction involves the insertion of a tissue expander deep to the pectoralis major. The expander is a silicone bag connected to a valve that is placed subcutaneously. The bag is filled gradually with saline by injecting percutaneously into the valve. Over a period of weeks the tissues can be stretched to accommodate a silastic implant of the size and shape to match the other breast. The implant is inserted at a second operation. An alternative form of expander has an expandable bag within a silicone gel prosthesis. There is no need for a second procedure other than the minor one of removing the valve once the inflation is completed.

Expander techniques are suitable for women with relatively small breasts that are not ptotic. The match between the sides is good when the woman is dressed, but the reconstructed side tends to be firmer than the natural side and therefore does not move in a realistic manner when the woman is undressed.

Myocutaneous flaps

When the breast is so large that tissue expansion is likely to be unsuccessful, muscle and skin can be moved from elsewhere to reconstruct the breast. Two flaps are in common use – the latissimus dorsi flap (Fig. 5.3) and the transverse rectus abdominus flap. Both have the disadvantage that additional scarring is left elsewhere. In the case of the latissimus dorsi flap this is on the back, while with the rectus abdominus flap it is on the lower abdomen. The muscle is kept attached to its neurovascular pedicle and is moved into position with the overlying skin.

The particular advantage of the latissimus dorsi flap is that it is robust and is unlikely to fail. The particular drawback is that a silastic implant is still needed. The transverse rectus abdominis flap is more prone to

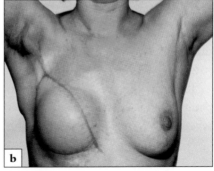

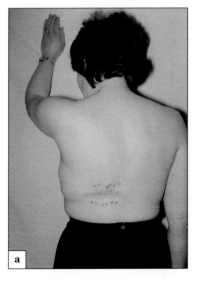

Figure 5.3. A latissimus dorsi reconstruction. (a) Residual scarring on the back. (b) Note the elliptical scar on the breast. Nipple reconstruction can be performed subsequently.

complications and cannot be carried out if the patient has extensive previous abdominal scarring. It is relatively contraindicated in smokers and the obese. Its major advantage is that it does not require a silastic implant and gives a very natural ptosis in most cases.

Free rectus flaps

Some plastic surgeons carry out the reconstruction using free rectus flaps. In these, the muscle is completely detached from its blood supply and the blood vessels are reimplanted using microvascular techniques. It is rarely necessary to carry out a free flap procedure to obtain a good cosmetic result.

Complications of reconstruction

For a number of years there has been intermittent bad publicity regarding silastic implants. It has been suggested that they are carcinogenic and more commonly that they give rise to connective tissue disorders. The current evidence does not show any increase in malignant disease or collagen disorders in patients with implants. The problems that occur are local. In the early stages, infection is a possibility and results in the prosthesis having to be removed. Later, the most common problem is capsular contraction. The prosthesis is surrounded by a capsule that contracts, which makes the prosthesis hard, spherical and painful. The only useful treatment is removal of the prosthesis and capsule. If the patient so wishes, a new prosthesis can be inserted.

The initial result of reconstruction is not always satisfactory and the patient must be warned before the process begins that it might require several revision operations before it is right.

RADIOTHERAPY

Like surgery, radiotherapy is principally used for the control of local disease. It has a lesser, though important, role in the management of metastatic disease, particularly in bone where it is very effective in controlling pain. Radiation is measured in 'grays' (1 Gy =100 rads) and the typical dose for breast cancer is between 50 and 60 Gy.

External beam radiation

The most common form of radiation used is external beam radiation, which employs high-energy X-rays generated by a linear accelerator. Radiation produces cell death by generation within the tissues of free radicals that damage the DNA. Normal tissues are affected as well as cancer cells, but normal cells have better DNA repair mechanisms and so can recover more quickly. To minimize the effects on normal tissue while producing cell kill in the cancer, the total dose that is required is given in small fractions spread out over 20–25 days. Fields are applied from different directions to reduce the radiation exposure of normal tissue. The fields are arranged so that the beams of radiation intersect at the tumour-bearing area, which therefore receives an additive dose of radiation. After general irradiation of the breast, some patients are given further doses focussed on the area from which the tumour was removed. This is known as a booster dose.

Computer-aided planning of the fields is needed to ensure that vital structures do not receive a damaging dose of radiation. Care must be taken to avoid the heart and lungs as far as possible.

The skin lies within the radiation field. Modern high-energy equipment is relatively sparing of the skin, but some effect inevitably occurs. Patients experience mild 'sunburn' that can be relieved symptomatically with bland preparations such as calamine lotion or E45 cream. The area must be treated gently and care must be taken with washing and bathing. Occasionally, the reaction is more severe. The radiotherapists prescribe mild corticosteroid ointments if needed.

Brachytherapy

An alternative approach to radiotherapy is the insertion of radioactive wires into the area to be irradiated. This is sometimes used for large primary tumours or for local recurrence after mastectomy that is not amenable to surgical excision. In the operating room, special thin tubes are inserted into the area to be treated. The patient is returned to the ward and the radioactive source then loaded into the tubes using special machinery that allows the material to be handled remotely, thus reducing the risk to the staff.

ADJUVANT THERAPY

One of the most important advantages in the management of breast cancer has been the introduction of adjuvant therapy. It is known that even when no metastases can be detected at the time of presentation, patients go on to develop distant disease, so undetectable micro-metastases must be present at the time of primary treatment. Adjuvant therapy is given to eliminate or control those micro-metastases. Initially, adjuvant therapy was thought to be effective only for those women who had prognostic factors that indicated a high risk of recurrence (e.g. involved lymph nodes). The Early Breast Cancer Trialists Collaborative Group carried out overviews of all the adjuvant therapy trials that have been published, and it is now apparent that the relative risk reduction achieved by adjuvant therapy is the same for all patients. Obviously, the higher the actual risk of recurrence, the greater is the absolute risk reduction brought about by treatment. The overview has also produced further evidence on what constitutes a high risk of recurrence and so the criteria for using adjuvant therapy have been altered. In each case, a balance has to be struck between the benefits to be obtained from adjuvant therapy and the side effects that it produces.

There are two categories of adjuvant therapy – hormonal therapy and chemotherapy. In broad terms, hormonal therapy is used in post-menopausal women and chemotherapy in premenopausal women, although there are exceptions to the rule. Some evidence indicates that premenopausal women with oestrogen-receptor positive tumours may benefit from ovarian ablation (surgical or medical), while younger post-menopausal women with oestrogen-receptor negative tumours may be offered chemotherapy.

Adjuvant therapy is maintained for varying lengths of time. Chemotherapy is usually given for 6 months as there does not appear to be any benefit in continuing it for longer. Tamoxifen (see below) is usually given for 5 years, and trials are in progress to determine whether longer treatment is better. Goserelin produces a medical ovarian ablation and has been given for 2 years in one trial. The long-term results are awaited.

Hormone therapy

About 60% of breast cancers display oestrogen and/or progesterone receptors, and these tumours appear to be dependent on hormones for growth and any interference with the hormonal milieu results in slowing the growth of the tumour. As all tumours are in a dynamic balance between cell division and cell death, if cell division is slowed or stopped the tumour regresses as a result of continued cell death. In general, tumours that are likely to respond to one form of hormone therapy are likely to respond to all forms of hormone therapy (Fig. 5.4). Tumours that relapse on one form of hormone therapy have around a 30% chance of responding to second-line therapy.

Tamoxifen

Tamoxifen is the mainstay of first-line endocrine therapy at present. It is a corticosteroid molecule that binds to the oestrogen receptor and has in some tissues a partial oestrogen agonist effect. In the breast it acts as a competitive inhibitor of oestrogen. It has been used for breast cancer since the mid-1970s and in advanced disease gives a 60% response rate in receptor-positive tumours. A small percentage of oestrogen receptor-negative tumours also respond, but the mechanism of this is unclear. Tamoxifen does appear to have anti-tumour properties that are unrelated to its anti-oestrogen effect, but it is also possible that some of the receptor-negative tumours that respond are, in fact, incorrectly reported as receptor negative.

Tamoxifen has an excellent side effect and toxicity profile. The major side effects relate to menstrual irregularity and hot flushes in premenopausal women. Visual side effects occur in a very small number

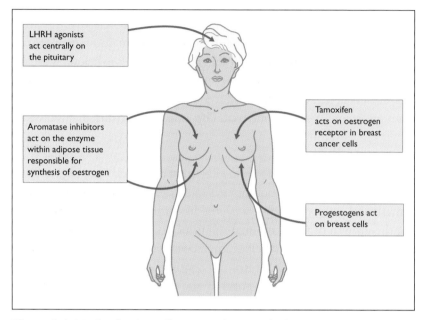

LHRH agonists act centrally on the pituitary

Aromatase inhibitors act on the enzyme within adipose tissue responsible for synthesis of oestrogen

Tamoxifen acts on oestrogen receptor in breast cancer cells

Progestogens act on breast cells

Figure 5.4. Mode of action of hormone therapies for breast cancer.

of patients and necessitate the cessation of treatment. Some patients complain of excessive weight gain. As a result of its partial agonist action, tamoxifen leads to an increased bone mineral density and to improved lipid profiles in postmenopausal women. Long-term use (over 10 years) is associated with endometrial hypertrophy and an increased incidence of endometrial carcinoma.

Tamoxifen has been shown to be effective as an adjuvant therapy, and in postmenopausal node-positive women results in an absolute survival advantage of 10% at 10 years. It reduces the risk of a woman developing a contralateral breast cancer by 30%. Trials have, therefore, been established to examine its role as a prophylactic agent in women with a high risk of developing breast cancer. The American trial has closed to recruitment, but the British and European trials are still recruiting. The effectiveness of tamoxifen as a prophylactic agent remains in doubt.

Aromatase inhibitors

In premenopausal women the ovaries are the main source of oestrogen, but in postmenopausal women oestrogen is produced in the peripheral adipose tissue from precursors from the adrenal glands. The enzyme concerned is called aromatase. Inhibition of aromatase, therefore, results in a reduction in the levels of circulating oestrogen.

Whereas tamoxifen acts as a competitive inhibitor of oestrogen, the aromatase inhibitors reduce the amount of oestrogen available to the tumour. The first of the useful aromatase inhibitors was aminoglutethimide. In addition to inhibiting oestrogen production this also inhibits the production of the glucocorticoids, so hydrocortisone has to be given with it unless a low dose is used. Newer aromatase inhibitors such as anastrazole (Arimidex) do not have a significant effect on the glucocorticoids.

Aromatase inhibitors are not effective in premenopausal women.

Progestogens

The effectiveness of the progestogens is similar to that of the other hormone therapies. Medroxyprogesterone acetate and megestrol acetate have been used, but only the latter is still in vogue. It is usually used as a third-line of therapy after relapse on aromatase inhibitors. A response rate of about 30% can be expected in these circumstances.

The major side effect of the progestogens is weight gain, which partly results from an increased appetite; the drugs can usefully be prescribed in the palliative setting to patients who complain of anorexia.

Luteinizing hormone releasing hormone agonists

Luteinizing hormone releasing hormone (LHRH) is released by the hypothalamus and stimulates the release of luteinizing hormone and follicle-stimulating hormone by the anterior pituitary. This in turn stimulates the ovaries. Drugs that mimic the action of LHRH are LHRH agonists. When they are given in depot form so that luteinizing-hormone release is permanently stimulated, they lead to exhaustion of the pituitary, which then ceases to produce luteinizing hormone and follicle-stimulating hormone. Since the ovaries are no longer stimu-lated, the levels of oestrogen and progesterone fall and, in effect, a medical oophorectomy is achieved. Depot goserelin is used in clinical practice for the treatment of advanced breast cancer. It has been used in trials as an adjuvant treatment.

Surgical ablation

The earliest hormonal therapy was surgical ablation of the ovaries (Beatson from Glasgow first reported this as being effective in 1896).The usual response rate was 30% as in the early years the tumours that were hormone dependent could not be identified. Patients who relapsed after a successful response to oophorectomy were then subjected to adrena-lectomy or hypophysectomy. A 30% response rate was again expected.

Drug therapy has largely replaced surgical ablation, with goserelin acting as a medical oophorectomy and aromatase inhibitors acting as a medical adrenalectomy.

Chemotherapy

Chemotherapeutic agents are essentially cell poisons that act in a vari-ety of ways to arrest cell growth or bring about cell death. As is the case with radiotherapy, they affect normal cells as well as malignant cells. As with radiotherapy, the normal cells recover more quickly than can the malignant cells. Advantage is taken of this by giving chemotherapy intermittently (usually every 3–4 weeks). By the time the next dose of chemotherapy is given the normal cells have recov-ered, but the malignant cells have not, and thus there is an incremen-tal loss of malignant cells as the chemotherapy proceeds.

Unlike radiotherapy, chemotherapy is systemic and affects all parts of the body. Cells that are dividing are more susceptible to the effects of chemotherapy, so tissues that have a high percentage of dividing cells (gastrointestinal epithelium, bone marrow) are more likely to sustain damage. The side effects of chemotherapy are related to this.

The principle side effects experienced by patients who receive chemotherapy used for breast cancer are nausea and vomiting, hair loss and a reduced white blood cell count. With some of the common regimens side effects are unlikely. When nausea is the major problem the symptoms can usually be controlled by anti-emetics. In severe cases, dexamethasone may be used. The white blood cell count must be carefully monitored and if the levels do fall the next dose of chemotherapy may be reduced or delayed.

High-dose chemotherapy that requires marrow rescue by bone marrow transplant or marrow-stimulating agents is under investigation in a number of studies. So far, there is no evidence that the extra benefit achieved outweighs the much higher incidence of side effects.

DISCUSSION

TG I have a question about radical versus local excision. I can understand the explanation here about the varying needs of patients and how certain factors affect what type of surgery is required. However, many patients would still prefer to have less-invasive surgery. If you felt that a mastectomy was indicated would you press for it without considering the patient's opinion?

SJL If the prognostic factors suggest that early recurrence is likely after conservative treatment, I would certainly press for the patient to accept a mastectomy. Clearly, it is important to explain carefully why a mastectomy is the better option. If the patient continues to want conservation after careful discussion, I would respect her wishes, but I would wish to be clear that she understood that she was placing herself at greater risk of local recurrence.

TG Do you think that this area of patient concern is important and how can we facilitate this area of pre-operative counselling? Is it for primary care to develop, or is it only relevant to secondary care?

SJL I think this area of counselling is extremely important. The breast care nurses play a vital role, but the patient should have access to a variety of informed advisors. The primary care team is likely to know the patient better and to have a deeper understanding of the reasons behind her concerns. The hospital team probably has a better understanding of the disease. Both perspectives are needed if the patient is to be given the best advice. This requires good communication between the two groups, particularly when the decision is not straightforward.

CT Often GPs are asked their opinion regarding reconstructive surgery, and whether patients should have this at the time of their original surgery, or after an interval. Is there any difference and does reconstruction make follow-up and detection of any recurrence more difficult?

SJL I have always been an advocate of immediate reconstruction. Survival and recurrence are not affected by the reconstruction and there seems to be no justification for a delay. There is no reason why reconstruction should make it more difficult to detect recurrence. It is sometimes more difficult to obtain a good cosmetic result with immediate reconstruction, but this can usually be corrected at a second operation. If a woman is uncertain about having reconstruction, I advise her to wait. It can be carried out as a delayed procedure whenever she decides she would like it.

TG What about radiotherapy and adjuvant systemic therapy? It would seem that some centres opt for multiple therapy, and therefore combine both. Is there any logic behind this? This is the time that most patients seek support from their GP and it is sometimes difficult to know what to say to them.

SJL One of the problems is that new evidence is accumulating all the time and treatment protocols change as a result. Whenever breast-conserving surgery is carried out it is common practice to give radiotherapy, which has been consistently shown to reduce the rate of local recurrence. Adjuvant systemic therapy is aimed at reducing metastatic disease and prolonging survival. Clearly, the two roles overlap but they are distinct and both forms of therapy need to be given. The indications for adjuvant therapy are extending all the time and you should ask for an explanation if a new patient does not receive adjuvant therapy. There is growing evidence that some patients benefit from radiotherapy even after a mastectomy and this may result in a prolongation of survival as well as a reduction in local recurrence.

Once again, the reasons for any treatment plan should be fully discussed with the patient.

CHAPTER SUMMARY

- The two-fold aim of treatment is the control of local disease and the prevention of distant disease.
- Surgery remains the mainstay of local control, but adjuvant radiotherapy is often indicated for optimum control.
- Breast conservation is sometimes contraindicated; in such cases breast reconstruction may be considered.
- Adjuvant hormone therapy or chemotherapy is given to reduce the chance of distant recurrence.

chapter 6

The management of early breast cancer

FACTORS THAT INFLUENCE TREATMENT DECISIONS

Patients with breast cancer are individuals and each patient's treatment should be tailored to her individual needs and to the nature of her tumour. The concept of a single 'correct' treatment for breast cancer is no longer tenable and the many available guidelines on treatment must be applied with discretion. The evidence on breast cancer treatment changes rapidly and it is necessary to modify the recommended treatment plans as new information becomes available. Nevertheless, certain underlying principles apply and in this chapter these are outlined and illustrated by considering 'typical' cases of breast cancer.

The treatment plan for an individual patient depends on *patient factors* and *tumour factors*.

Patient factors

The most important patient factor is what the patient wants. The patient's involvement in the decision making process may influence her psychological response to her disease and treatment (more fully considered in Chapter 8). Other factors that may influence the treatment include the patient's age and menopausal status.

Tumour characteristics

The appropriate treatment for a given patient depends on the predicted behaviour of the tumour. If it can be predicted that a tumour has a high likelihood of recurrence after breast conservation, it is wiser to advise mastectomy. When the development of metastatic disease can be predicted, adjuvant therapy is indicated.

If the invasive tumour is associated with extensive ductal carcinoma *in situ* (DCIS) or with vascular or lymphatic invasion, it is more likely to recur locally if treated conservatively. Larger, Grade 3 tumours also have an increased chance of recurrence, particularly in younger women.

The presence of lymph node metastases is one of the strongest predictors of distant metastases.

TREATMENT

Breast conservation

When the tumour is suitable for conservation (see Table 5.1) and the patient is in agreement, the initial procedure is wide local excision of the tumour and removal of axillary lymph nodes. Controversy surrounding both of these procedures has occurred in the past, but it is now agreed that excision of the breast lump with a clear margin of tissue is adequate. There is no need for larger procedures such as quadrantectomy. Radiotherapy is needed after tumour excision to prevent recurrence.

Treatment of the axilla

The correct axillary procedure is still unclear. The nodes have to be removed to determine whether they are involved. If they are, this affects decisions on further treatment. Attempts are being made to devise ways of deciding on the lymph node status without carrying out an axillary clearance. The most promising of these is sentinel node biopsy, the underlying concept of which is simple. The region of the tumour in the breast is infiltrated with either a dye or a radioisotope. This marker is taken up and appears in the lymph nodes. The lowest lymph node to contain the marker is excised and submitted to histology. If this node is clear no further surgery is necessary, but if it is involved the axilla must be cleared. Proof that this procedure is useful clinically is still awaited.

Mastectomy

When the tumour is unsuitable for conservation, a mastectomy must be recommended. If a patient does undergo mastectomy, it is possible to carry out reconstruction either at the time of mastectomy or at any later time convenient to the patient. Radiotherapy is not routinely used after mastectomy, but it may be prescribed in younger women with large, high-grade tumours, or major lymph node involvement.

CASE STUDIES

Case study 6.1

A 55-year-old postmenopausal woman presented with a carcinoma and it was treated by wide local excision and axillary clearance. On histology the tumour was described as a 20 mm, Grade 2 invasive ductal carcinoma and is oestrogen-receptor positive. The 12 lymph nodes examined were found to be free from tumour.

Discussion

SJL This is a straightforward case. The tumour is suitable for treatment by conservation. The patient is postmenopausal and the tumour is oestrogen-receptor positive. She is an ideal candidate for adjuvant tamoxifen.

TG You've mentioned grade again. Does that influence your decision on treatment?

SJL The simple answer is yes, but the detail is complicated. If the
tumour is Grade 3, I would more probably consider mastectomy,
but the final decision would depend on the size of the tumour
and the age of the patient.

CT What would you do if this tumour were oestrogen-receptor negative?

SJL As this patient is postmenopausal and node negative I would still
put her on tamoxifen. Her risk of recurrence is moderate rather
than high and the absolute improvement in survival as a result
of chemotherapy is not great. I do not believe it warrants the
potential side effects. There is some evidence that tamoxifen is
effective to some extent even in tumours that are oestrogen-receptor negative. The side effects of tamoxifen in postmenopausal
women are unlikely to be severe.

CT How long would you continue the adjuvant tamoxifen?

SJL The current routine is 5 years, but clinical trials are underway to
establish whether a longer duration of treatment produces greater
benefit.

TG I take it you refer her for radiotherapy?

SJL Yes. I believe the recurrence rate without radiotherapy is unac-
ceptably high.

Case study 6.2

A 42-year-old premenopausal woman has undergone wide local excision and axillary clearance for a 30 mm, Grade 3 invasive ductal carcinoma of no special type. Vascular invasion is seen, but the tumour is oestrogen-receptor positive. The excision margins are clear. Three of 15 lymph nodes contain metastatic breast cancer.

Discussion

SJL This is a much more difficult case than case study 6.1. The prognosis is not good with a high risk of distant metastases, but the size, grade and vascular invasion indicate a major risk of local recurrence. As a consequence of this, I would discuss the need for a mastectomy with the patient. She requires adjuvant chemotherapy on several grounds, particularly the nodal status.

TG Does it not cause problems to go back to the patient after she has had surgery and tell her that she needs another operation?

SJL Yes it does, but even core biopsies do not necessarily give you all the information that is needed to decide that the tumour is likely to recur after conservative therapy. There is really no alternative to accepting that a certain number of patients will need a second operation.

HD We make a point of warning the patients of this possibility during the preoperative counselling.

CT Are there any other factors that would lead you to suggest that a patient needed a mastectomy?

SJL If there is extensive DCIS associated with the invasive tumour, the incidence of recurrence is high. I would also favour a mastectomy if multifocal disease was present, but this is often detected preoperatively on mammography. Some surgeons regard involvement of the excision margin with tumour as an indication for a mastectomy, but I would tend to suggest a wider excision to clear the margins.

TG You specify that three lymph nodes are involved. Is there any significance to the number of involved lymph nodes?

SJL The prognosis does depend on the number of lymph nodes that are involved. The division is rather artificial, but the prognosis is regarded as being poor if more than four nodes are involved. If more than 10 nodes are involved the prognosis is very poor. There are no hard and fast rules, but patients with 1–3 nodes involved tend to be treated with standard chemotherapy regimens, such as cyclophosphamide, methotrexate and 5-fluorouracil. When more than four nodes are involved, regimens that contain anthracyclines (e.g. doxorubicin) are often used. There are trials underway on high-dose chemotherapy for patients with more than 10 involved nodes. These regimens result in severe marrow suppression and must include marrow rescue using cytokines or autologous bone marrow transplant.

CT For how long is the adjuvant treatment given?

SJL The chemotherapy usually lasts for 6 months, but the patient would then be put on tamoxifen for at least 5 years. The optimal duration of tamoxifen therapy is still being investigated.

Case study 6.3

A 60-year-old woman has an area of microcalcification detected at breast screening. A core biopsy confirms a diagnosis of DCIS.

CT Is there any difference in your approach to DCIS and lobular carcinoma *in situ* (LCIS)?

SJL Very definitely – DCIS is a genuine pre-invasive cancer and it is assumed that a high percentage progress to invasive tumour if left untreated. On the other hand, LCIS is a marker for the risk that the woman may develop breast cancer at a later time. Curiously, they are as likely to develop cancer in the opposite breast as in the affected breast, with a 15% risk in each breast at 10 years.

There is still doubt about the best treatment for DCIS. In the past, all women with DCIS were treated by mastectomy, which was effective and resulted in almost a 100% cure rate. The belief is developing that this is over-treatment and there is evidence that wide local excision and radiotherapy is effective for localized DCIS. The results of trials of surgery alone or along with tamoxifen are awaited. The risk of further disease developing is higher if the DCIS is high grade and multifocal. In these cases mastectomy is still advised.

CT How do you know when the disease is multifocal?

SJL Often there is an indication on the mammogram, but sometimes it is not until the histology is available that the cancer is found to be multifocal. The patient who undergoes wide local excision must always be counselled that further surgery might prove to be necessary.

TG You haven't told us what you do for LCIS.

SJL As LCIS is a risk factor for the development of breast cancer, rather than a pre-malignant condition, it is more rational to keep the patient under close observation with annual mammography rather than to carry out further surgery. If a patient does insist on further surgery, the only logical approach is to carry out a bilateral mastectomy. There is no indication for unilateral mastectomy.

CT Presumably, the microcalcification is impalpable; how do you identify it at operation?

SJL The area has to be marked preoperatively. We usually insert a marking wire under stereotactic radiological control. At operation we follow the wire to the correct area. If there is an impalpable mass rather than an area of microcalcification, it can be identified by ultrasound scan and the overlying skin can be marked instead of inserting a wire. A radiograph is taken of the excised tissue to confirm that the suspicious lesion has been removed.

Case study 6.4

A 48-year-old woman has been on HRT for 5 years. She presents with a breast cancer and it is decided to carry out wide local excision and axillary clearance to be followed by radiotherapy. She attends the surgery to ask what she should do about her HRT.

Discussion

TG This is one of the questions that I find very difficult. Should she stop her HRT or not?

SJL I agree, this is very difficult. Let's review the facts. There is evidence that patients who have been on HRT for more than 5 years have an increased risk of developing breast cancer. The actual increase in risk is not great, with the relative risk of 'ever users' of HRT being calculated at 1.023 as compared to 'never users' in a recent overview. What is not known is what the effect of HRT is on diagnosed breast cancer. Small studies that have been carried out have not produced any evidence of a worse prognosis for women with breast cancer being treated with HRT. Nevertheless, it is not possible to give an absolute guarantee that HRT does not affect the outcome.

I take a pragmatic approach. When the woman is taking HRT for symptom relief rather than for the prevention of osteoporosis or cardiovascular disease, I suggest that she stop HRT to see what happens. If her symptoms become intolerable I then suggest re-starting HRT, although I warn her that I could not guarantee that it would not worsen her prognosis. Curiously, if tamoxifen is given with the HRT, it does not prevent HRT relieving the symptoms. Progestogens such as megestrol acetate are effective in some women.

If the reason the patient is on HRT is for treatment or prophylaxis of osteoporosis or cardiovascular disease, alternative therapies are now available. These are said not to have any effect on the breast tissue, but there is no clinical trial evidence to support the view that these treatments are safer.

Case study 6.5

A 76-year-old woman suffers from ischaemic heart disease. She has had two previous myocardial infarctions, the last being 9 months ago. She is in atrial fibrillation and has angina on climbing a flight of stairs.

She is currently on diuretics to control her cardiac failure and is on warfarin, which her cardiologist says should not be stopped. She attends with a probable carcinoma of the right breast.

Discussion

CT This woman is clearly unfit for surgery. Is there any point in referring her to the breast clinic or should we just prescribe tamoxifen on the assumption that she has breast cancer?

SJL I must say that I prefer to have a definitive diagnosis before I start any form of treatment. If she is referred to the clinic we can confirm the diagnosis using the triple assessment. The fact that she is anticoagulated does not prevent a fine needle aspiration. I agree that she is not an ideal candidate for surgery and if her tumour is oestrogen-receptor positive tamoxifen would be the treatment of choice. Care has to be taken with her anticoagulation as tamoxifen potentiates the effect of warfarin, so her warfarin dose has to be adjusted. If her tumour is oestrogen-receptor negative or does not respond to tamoxifen, I would ask for anaesthetic opinion on whether she could be made fit for operation.

CHAPTER SUMMARY

- The treatment must be tailored to the individual patient and depends on the characteristics of the patient and the tumour.
- Breast conservation is not always possible.
- Axillary surgery is indicated for accurate staging of the disease. Newer approaches may reduce the extent of axillary surgery that is needed.

chapter 7

The follow-up of patients with breast cancer

The problems of how often a woman with breast cancer should be followed up, who should do it and for how long it should be done are unclear. There is a long tradition of follow-up being carried out by the specialists, with many women attending the surgeon and the clinical oncologist for many years. An expectation has developed among the general public that this is the appropriate method for effective patient care. There is little evidence that regular specialist follow-up has any effect on disease progression. Indeed, even in the presence of intensive follow-up, the patient usually detects recurrences herself between routine visits.

Perhaps we should not look for a single 'correct' approach to the question of follow-up. Different approaches may be needed for different patients. It is inherently unlikely that a patient with a small, well-differentiated tumour of good prognosis needs the same follow-up regimen as a patient with an aggressive tumour. Some patients may like the security of attending the hospital, while others may prefer to be seen by their GP. If follow-up is to occur in hospital, an argument can be made for it to be carried out by specialist nurses. The reality of hospital follow-up is that the patient is likely to be seen by a junior member of the medical team who has not seen her before and is unlikely to see her again because of the rotation of junior staff. A permanent nurse practitioner is more likely to form a continuing relationship with the patient, which will give better psychological support and make the detection of subtle changes more probable.

RECURRENCE IN PATIENTS WITH BREAST CANCER

The probability of recurrence is dependent on the prognostic features of the cancer and the use or not of adjuvant therapy. Whatever the overall prognosis of the tumour, the incidence of recurrence is higher in the earlier years after diagnosis, although recurrence can happen even after many years of disease-free survival. As a result of the higher incidence in the earlier years it is common practice to offer intensive follow-up in the first 2 years after diagnosis and reduce the frequency as time goes on. Although the disease can recur after many years, the incidence of recurrence after 5 years is low and it is common practice to stop routine follow-up after 5 or 10 years.

WHY IS FOLLOW-UP CARRIED OUT?

There are three valid reasons for the follow-up patients:

- First is the belief that the early detection of recurrent disease results in an improvement in the patient's chances of survival.
- Second is that regular follow-up provides psychological support to the patient.
- Third is that it provides data for audit and research.

The underlying assumption behind the first reason does not stand up to scrutiny. No evidence indicates that treating metastatic disease earlier than the point at which it becomes clinically apparent has any effect on the survival of the patient. If earlier treatment does not alter the outcome, screening merely serves to make the patient aware of her problem for a longer time. In practice, it is rare for the recurrence to be detected in the preclinical stage.

In the case of breast cancer, the exception to this negative view of the value of follow-up is the detection by regular mammography of recurrence within the conserved breast or of a new primary in the contralateral breast. No empirical data acquired from well-designed and conducted studies exist to indicate how often this mammography should be carried out to improve the patient's chance of survival. Current consensus recommendations are annually for the conserved breast and biannually for the contralateral breast.

Although follow-up has not been shown to be effective, some patients obtain a sense of security from being seen regularly. These patients may be reluctant to stop attending, even after 10 years, and in these cases follow-up does provide psychological support. For other patients the follow-up acts as a reminder that they have been treated for breast cancer. They find this very stressful and have a period of increased anxiety leading up to the attendance at the clinic. They may have a marked sense of relief following the clinic attendance, but this wide swing of emotions may be a source of psychological stress. These patients might be better served by not being seen regularly. It is not easy to separate the two groups so that a different strategy can be applied to each. Some patients who experience high levels of anxiety claim to experience the highest level of psychological support from the follow-up.

It is clearly important to have accurate outcome data for research and audit, but creative solutions are required to obtain this data via a less resource-intensive method and in a way less traumatic to the patient than regular visits to the clinic.

WHO SHOULD CARRY OUT THE FOLLOW-UP?

Studies that compare follow-up by the primary care team with follow-up by the hospital have shown no advantage for those patients followed up by the hospital. The studies are not as conclusive as they appear because only those patients who were happy to enter either arm of the studies were selected. Thus, a patient who preferred to be followed up by the hospital was followed by the hospital, which may have produced bias in the oncological outcome and certainly produced bias in the psychological outcome.

Other studies suggest that patients do not believe that the primary care team knows enough about breast cancer to carry out the follow-up.

Of course, one practical interpretation is that patients should be allowed to select their own pattern of follow-up.

CHAPTER SUMMARY

- The efficacy of follow-up of patients with breast cancer has not yet been proved.
- Regular mammography is currently recommended for all women who have been treated for breast cancer.
- There may be a role for follow-up in the psychological support of patients, but for some patients the process in itself provokes anxiety.
- Women should be encouraged to select the pattern of follow-up that is most congenial to themselves.

chapter 8

Managing the psychological consequences of breast cancer

As has already been noted, many patients suffer from psychological morbidity as a result of breast disease. A widespread fear of breast cancer is fuelled by the media so that any woman who develops a symptom in her breast is likely to be extremely anxious. The level of anxiety in women who actually have benign disease is as high prior to diagnosis as that of women who are subsequently diagnosed as having breast cancer. When breast conservation was originally popularized, the expectation was that it would result in a reduced level of psychological morbidity. This has proved not to be the case. The type of psychological distress tends to be different, but the incidence is the same. Women who have undergone mastectomy tend to develop depression; women who have undergone breast conservation tend to develop anxiety. The level of morbidity can be altered – this seems to depend on the approach of the medical staff to the patient. Patient-centred approaches that respect the individuality of the patient appear to result in lower levels of morbidity.

Psychological distress may develop at any time during the trajectory of the illness and it is important that it is actively sought during follow-up. The patient may well not bring psychological symptoms to the attention of her doctors, either because she thinks they are 'natural' for someone in her situation or else because she thinks such symptoms are not relevant to her medical care.

The four important components to managing the patient's psychological distress are given in the box.

MANAGING THE PATIENT'S PSYCHOLOGICAL DISTRESS

- Shorten the period of uncertainty as much as possible
- Encourage the patient to be involved in decision making
- Give an adequate level of information in understandable terms
- Spend time with the patient and her relatives

SHORTENING THE PERIOD OF UNCERTAINTY AS MUCH AS POSSIBLE

The period from discovery of a breast symptom until the establishment of a firm diagnosis should be as short as possible. Logistic problems with meeting this aim arise because of the large numbers of women with breast symptoms. It can be very difficult to decide who has a problem that needs further investigation and who can be simply reassured. Often the most anxious patient is the one who is least likely to have a problem, but needs referral before she can be reassured.

Once the patient is seen by the breast clinic every effort must be made to reach a diagnosis as quickly as possible. As has been discussed earlier, it is now possible in many cases to give a firm diagnosis at the first visit.

ENCOURAGE THE PATIENT TO BE INVOLVED IN THE DECISION MAKING

The realization is increasing that respect for the patient's autonomy means that the patient must be involved in the decisions about her treatment. Furthermore, evidence indicates that involvement of the patient in the decision making results in a reduction in the incidence of severe psychological morbidity. The reason for this is unclear. Fallowfield's study suggests that it is the underlying attitude of the surgeon that is important. Patients who were treated by a surgeon who preferred to offer a choice of treatments had less psychological morbidity than those who were treated by surgeons who did not offer the patient any choice. However, this benefit persisted even when the surgeon who would normally offer choice was unable to do so. This suggested that the effect resulted from the surgeon's approach to the patient rather than from the choice itself.

To add further confusion, many patients with breast cancer do not want to take part in the decision-making process. In contrast to members of the general public who say that if they had breast cancer they would want to participate in decisions about the treatment, patients newly diagnosed with breast cancer express a preference for a more passive role. This tendency to transfer responsibility for decision making to the doctor becomes more marked after 2 years of follow-up after treatment.

It does appear that discussing the treatment with the patient and giving her the opportunity to be involved in the decisions, whether she takes it or not, helps to reduce psychological morbidity. This does mean that the patient must be given time to think over her options and reach an informed decision. Some patients reach a decision very quickly and are able to tell the surgeon what they want before they leave the first consultation. Others may need to go away and return on another occasion. Whatever approach the patient prefers, it is important that she realizes that her choice is not irrevocable and that she can change her mind at any time before the actual treatment is carried out.

In our practice, the breast-care nurse who has been present during the consultation arranges to visit the woman at home after 2–3 days. This gives the patient time to think things over and to discuss the situation with her friends and family. The home visit is preferable to another visit to the hospital as the patient has the psychological advantage of being in her own territory and therefore may feel more secure in her conversation with the breast care nurse.

When for oncological reasons only one line of treatment is rational, the patient can still be involved in the decision making if the facts are explained to them.

Of course, if the patient wishes to hand over all responsibility for the decision to the doctor, this is a valid exercise of autonomy and should be respected. The patient must be given the opportunity to hand over responsibility; the doctor must not assume it without being asked to do so, nor hold on to responsibility should the patient wish to reclaim it.

GIVING INFORMATION IN UNDERSTANDABLE TERMS

One of the persistent fallacies in education is the belief that because I have told somebody something they must have absorbed the information. There are many reasons for a failure to communicate, but one of the most important is a failure to present the information in a form that can be understood by the recipient. This usually means giving the message in simple terms, but may mean using appropriate technical explanations if the patient is capable of understanding them, and is willing to. It is as much a failure of communication to oversimplify the message for someone who is capable of understanding technicalities as it is to obscure the message in technical terms for someone without that background.

It is essential first of all to determine what the patient knows already and what she understands by the various words used by the doctor. If the word 'cancer' means inevitable, rapid and painful death to the patient, she will receive entirely the wrong message. This does not mean avoiding the word cancer; it does mean finding out exactly what the patient understands by what you say and correcting any misapprehensions during the conversation.

Simplification does not mean hiding the facts, but it may mean starting with a basic explanation of biology. By using diagrams and analogies, even quite complex ideas can be explained.

Written material can be useful in reinforcing the explanation that is given. Care must be taken to ensure that the literature is easily read – the reading age should be around 10–11 years if it is going to be understood by the majority of the readers. Anxiety results in an effective lowering of the reading age and if the leaflets are aimed at a higher reading age the patients struggle with them. Glossy, mass-produced material may not be as effective as more focussed locally prepared leaflets. It is good practice to give the patient material that is specific to their own condition and proposed treatment, rather than a general leaflet that might confuse them by discussing problems that they do not face.

Not all patients want the same level of information. It is important to listen to what the patient wants and not launch into a routine 'tutorial' on breast cancer, its consequences and its treatment. The emphasis should be on a dialogue with the patient and her supporters, rather than a monologue. The two-way trading of questions and answers ensures that the right level and amount of information is given. Information should not be forced on a patient who doesn't want it, any more than it should be withheld from a patient who does.

It is generally best if a relative or friend accompanies the patient, especially in the early consultations. The anxiety created by the diagnosis interferes with the patient's ability to listen to the explanations given and to recall them. A supporter may be able to remember more clearly and may also be able to ask more pertinent questions.

It is our practice in the breast clinic to have a breast-care nurse present during the consultation. She is then in a position to rehearse with the patient what has been said. This reiteration is repeated at the home visit.

We have conducted a study of the patients' needs for information and how they are met. Immediately after the diagnosis, patients tend to see the consultant as the major source of information with the breast-care nurse being regarded as a valuable adjunct. They find the leaflets issued by the breast unit helpful, but disappointingly do not turn to the primary care team as a resource (Fig. 8.1). At 2 years from diagnosis 60% of the patients still have unmet needs for information, but are unlikely to turn to any of the members of the primary care or specialist team. They tend to use the general media as their source. Given the inaccuracy of some media reports, this is a cause for concern (Fig. 8.2).

There is clearly a need for the care team to be proactive in finding out what information the patient wants and to attempt to give it.

The pattern of the type of information the patient is interested in fairly clear. The top three concerns for patients are 'Can the disease be cured?', 'How advanced is the disease?' and 'What does the treatment involve?'. Patients are much less concerned about other matters such as what effect the disease will have on their social life or their sexual activity. At 2 years from diagnosis they do start to be interested in whether their families are at risk, but the chance of cure and the extent of the disease remain their primary concerns.

SPEND TIME WITH THE PATIENT AND HER SUPPORTERS

If an adequate dialogue is to take place and the patient is to be involved in the decision-making process it is imperative that time is spent with the patient and her relatives and supporters. This is not so much a matter of chronological time as of perceived time. The setting of the conversation must be such that the patient feels there is no rush. This can be difficult to achieve in a busy clinic or surgery, so if necessary a special appointment must be made to allow an unhurried discussion. We do manage it in the course of the clinic by using a room that is

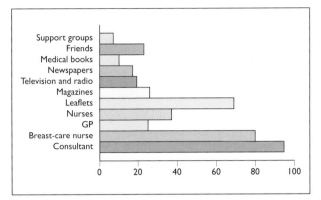

Figure 8.1.
Sources of
information:
newly diagnosed.

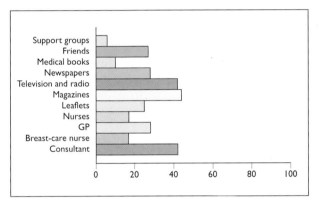

Figure 8.2.
Sources of
information:
follow-up.

dedicated to the purpose so that the rest of the clinic can proceed without interruption.

The offer of another meeting in the near future, after the patient has had time to digest what has been said also produces the perception of time being available. For many patients the offer of another meeting is sufficient in itself and the meeting does not take place. It is also important that the patient has easy access to a member of the team. Again, the majority of patients do not take advantage of the access. What reduces their anxiety is knowing that they can have another meeting if they feel need.

DISCUSSION

TG I agree that there is a need to refer patients as quickly as possible if malignancy is suspected, but how do we balance this against both not inducing too much anxiety and the need for the GP to be involved with the overall management and not simply as a point of referral?

SJL I think this dilemma highlights the role of the GP. The patient has to be referred for the diagnosis to be made, but the GP can begin the process of managing her anxiety at that point. An explanation of the reason for referral (to have the appropriate investigations carried out) and of the possible outcomes is useful. The patient should be given the opportunity to discuss her fears and to ask questions. If the GP is seen to be knowledgeable at this stage, it is likely that the patient will return for support in the future.

CT How can we improve the communication that occurs between the hospital and GP to maximize care while supporting the patient psychologically?

SJL We make a point of telephoning the GP whenever we make a diagnosis of breast cancer. It is also important that letters should be sent promptly and should contain relevant details of the proposed treatment.

HD The breast-care nurses can form a useful link. The patients are encouraged to telephone the breast-care nurse if there is a problem. The primary care team can also contact the breast-care nurses and may this easier than reaching a member of the medical staff. Since the breast care nurse is familiar with the routine of the unit, she is often able to answer the question that is being raised.

TG From what you describe, there is obviously a need for a breast-cancer liaison nurse. Where do you think the role of the practice nurse is in patient management?

HD The practice nurse has a potentially important role in supporting the patient. The women often feel comfortable talking to her and may bring her problems that they perceive as being too trivial to bring to the doctor. There is obviously a need for practice nurses to have appropriate training and knowledge.

SJL I think the emphasis should be on multiple sources of support so that the woman can find the support that she finds helpful.

TG Much is written in the lay press about complementary therapies, particularly in supporting patients in psychological distress. What is your view and do you think these therapies have a place?

SJL We probably should have had an entire chapter on this, or maybe a book. This is an aspect of the multiple sources of support and the patient finding for herself what is helpful to her. If a patient is interested to try complementary therapy I would encourage her. We do have a National Health Service unit locally that offers a wide range of complementary therapies. I think we have a responsibility to inform ourselves about complementary therapies so that we can hold an informed discussion with patients.

CHAPTER SUMMARY

- It is important to recognize psychological morbidity in patients with breast cancer. This requires active searching for psychological symptoms.
- The patient should be encouraged to be actively involved in decisions about her treatment.
- Information should be given to the patient and her supporters at an appropriate level and in appropriate terms.
- The most important element in giving support to patients is spending time with them.

chapter 9

Epilogue

Breast disease is a rapidly developing field. While the basic knowledge that underpins the understanding and approach to treatment adopted in this book is unlikely to change, it is certain that many of the details will change over the next few years. It is obviously impossible to predict exactly what those changes will be, but some informed guesses can be made about the direction in which those changes will occur.

BIOLOGY

It is likely that we will develop a better understanding of the molecular events that lead to the development of breast cancer. As the human genome becomes more clearly understood, it will become possible to identify the specific abnormalities that lead to changes in the breast epithelium. It will then be possible to test not only for familial genetic changes, but also for those that arise sporadically. At present, it is not possible on a routine basis to detect mutations, even in patients with a known family history. The technology may become available to allow significant mutations to be detected in women from the general population. This will alter the entire approach to screening and to prevention.

A less ambitious target is the selection of therapy for individual patients based on the prediction of response to various therapies from the molecular profile of the tumour. In its simplest form this is seen in the use of oestrogen-receptor status to predict the response to hormone therapy. There is already some indication that the response to chemotherapy can be predicted from the tumour's expression of *p53*. More detailed matrices of tumour characteristics against therapeutic response may be produced, which will eliminate the present blunderbuss approach to adjuvant therapy in particular, and identify those patients who will benefit from therapy.

PREVENTION

Better identification of women at risk of developing breast cancer will allow better targetted prevention campaigns. Eventually, the aim will be the introduction of gene therapy designed to correct the underlying genetic defect directly. This is still a long way off. Until then, chemoprevention using drugs that modify gene expression or cell differentiation will continue to be used. Currently, tamoxifen is the only candidate drug being tested, but others will be introduced.

DIAGNOSIS

Better imaging modalities may well be developed. Improvements in ultrasound scanning may increase both the ease of use and the discriminatory power. The quality of mammography is constantly improving. Eventually, all imaging modalities may be digitized and thus be amenable to computer analysis. The automation of film reading will not eliminate the need for radiologists, but may allow pre-screening so that only those films that are likely to show an abnormality will have to be read. This will be of major value in screening programmes.

Fine-needle aspiration cytology may be improved by the increased use of immunological markers that will improve the diagnostic accuracy and may give some predictive information to allow a more rational planning of therapy.

THERAPY

The principles of surgery are unlikely to change, although clearer indications for particular techniques are likely to emerge. Newer modalities such as microwaves are being tested as adjuncts to surgery, and may find a place in the procedure. Computed targetting for impalpable lesions may be developed and allow these lesions to be treated by minimally invasive techniques without the need for formal surgical excision.

There will be improvements in the drug treatment of breast cancer with newer hormonal and chemotherapeutic agents becoming available.

The major advances are likely to be in the area of gene therapy. At first, this will involve methods of ensuring that the tumour is more responsive to chemotherapeutic agents than normal tissue by the introduction of genes that regulate enzyme production. Eventually, the hope is that the genome of the tumour can be manipulated directly to repair the defect that renders the cell cancerous. This is still some way off and conventional therapy will be the mainstay of treatment for a long time.

PSYCHOLOGICAL SUPPORT

The current emphasis on psychological support for patients with breast disease will continue to grow. As our understanding of the psychological processes becomes more refined, so the management will become more focussed on the approach that is appropriate for a given woman. More attention will be turned to the needs of the family and significant others. There is an increasing awareness of the spiritual needs of patients who develop cancer. More information is needed in this area.

... AND SOME THINGS DON'T CHANGE

Whatever new developments occur, the fundamental need of a woman with breast symptoms is to meet a competent and caring practitioner with the necessary clinical and communication skills to diagnose her problem and manage it appropriately. A team approach is essential and is well established within specialist breast units. We must foster co-operation between the primary care team and the specialist team to provide genuine shared care. The patient must remain central to everything we do.

Recommended reading

- Baum M, Saunders C. *Breast Cancer: a guide for every woman.* Oxford: Oxford University Press; 1994.

- Cancer Research Campaign. *Breast Cancer Factsheet 6.* London: Cancer Research Campaign; 1991.

- Denton S. *Breast Cancer Nursing.* London: Chapman and Hall; 1996.

- Dixon M, Sainsbury R. *Handbook of Diseases of the Breast.* London: Churchill Livingstone; 1998.

- Dixon M. *ABC of Breast Diseases.* London: BMJ Publishing Group; 1997.

- Doyal L. *Women and Health Services.* Buckingham: Open University Press; 1998.

- Fallowfield LJ, Hall A, Maguire P *et al.* Psychological effects of being offered choice of surgery for breast cancer. *BMJ* 1994; 309: 448.

- Faulkner A, Maguire P. *Talking to Cancer Patients and their Relatives.* Oxford: Oxford University Press; 1994.

- McPherson A, Waller D. *Women's Health.* Oxford General Practice Series. Oxford: Oxford Medical Publications; 1997.

- NHSBSP. *NHS Breast Screening Programme Review.* Sheffield: NHSBSP; 1996.

- RCGP and OPCS. *Morbidity Statistics from General Practice 1991–92. RCGP and OPCS Fourth National Study.* London: HMSO; 1995.

Index